rary

New MRCPsych Paper I care 'apers

ng for you, wher

ıg the following cc

A Library, please

nped, unless re

ır one

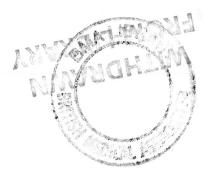

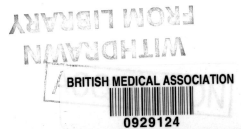

New MRCPsych Paper II Mock MCQ Papers

VELLINGIRI BADRAKALIMUTHU

MBBS, MRCPsych

Specialty Registrar in Old Age Psychiatry
PBL Tutor for CT1 and CT2 Psychiatry Trainees
Norfolk and Waveney Mental Health Foundation NHS Trust
Julian Hospital, Norwich

Foreword by

HUGO de WAAL

MD, FRCPsych

Lead Clinician for North Norfolk
Head of School, Postgraduate School of Psychiatry,
East of England Deanery
College Tutor, Norfolk and Waveney Psychiatric Training Scheme
Fellow, Higher Education Academy

Radcliffe Publishing
Oxford • New York

Radcliffe Publishing Ltd
18 Marcham Road
Abingdon
Oxon OX14 1AA
United Kingdom

www.radcliffe-oxford.com
Electronic catalogue and worldwide online ordering facility.

British Library Cataloguing in Publication Data

A catalogue record for this book is available from the British Library.

ISBN-13: 978 184619 395 8

The paper used for the text pages of this book
is FSC certified. FSC (The Forest Stewardship
Council) is an international network to promote
responsible management of the world's forests.

Mixed Sources
Product group from well-managed
forests and other controlled sources
www.fsc.org Cert no. SGS-COC-2482
© 1996 Forest Stewardship Council

FSC

Typeset by Pindar NZ, Auckland, New Zealand
Printed and bound by TJI Digital, Padstow, Cornwall, UK

Contents

Foreword

There aren't many books with a preface which contains an allusion to $E=MC^2$ and immediately go on to encourage a symbiotic relationship with a mould-forming kitchen sink (no matter how readily recognisable the latter is to anyone who ever studied relativity at University, or indeed anyone who ever revised for an exam). In fact, I would opine there is only the one. It could be understood as symptomatic for the breadth of Dr Badrakalimuthu's second MRCPsych preparation work. Once again tried and tested on the trainees in Norwich resulting in a pass percentage that continues to be higher than the national average, emphasising the completeness and thoroughness of the work.

This somewhat encyclopaedic feature immediately reminds one of the life and times of the legendary Oliver Goldsmith, who posthumously provided the motto to this book. Born in 1728 in Roscommon, Ireland, Mr Goldsmith's academic career started at the age of 16 at Trinity College, Dublin. After graduation (it is not quite clear in what topic of study) he became a tutor, but he was sacked after a quarrel. He tried to emigrate to America, but missed his ship: not as easily done as missing one's flight from Heathrow. His next project, studying law, was unwillingly shortened by gambling away the funds that were meant to sustain him. Sometime later he shows up on a walking tour through Flanders, having previously apparently studied medicine in Edinburgh and possibly Leiden (Holland). He wound his way on the roads as he did in academia, and meandered into Italy via France and Switzerland, earning his keep by playing the flute. Returning to London he blossomed into an author, playwright and poet and finally reached a position of fame.

One of his earliest works was entitled *Enquiry into the Present State of Polite Learning* (1759), in which he wrote:

> Does the poet paint the absurdities of the vulgar, then he is *low*; does he

exaggerate the features of folly, to render it more ridiculous, he is then *very low*. In short, they have proscribed the comic or satirical muse from every walk but high life, which, though abounding in fools as well as the humblest station, is by no means so fruitful in absurdity.

This brings us neatly to that lofty institution, which sets the curriculum and exam questions you are assumed to be preparing for: you may at times view those questions absurd to a degree, deemed lamentably absent by Goldsmith in 'high life'. If so, it might be useful to remind yourself that throughout your professional career the absurdities of the vulgar are never thus: no matter what 'station' our patients inhabit, the vulgar are never vulgar, their problems never absurd and fools are few and far between. It could therefore be argued that, whilst revising for the exam, your necessary obsession with the absurd constitutes somewhat of a professional desensitisation: once you are versant in the questions and answers contained in the Royal College's membership examinations, there won't be much on the face of this earth that would strike you as extraordinary, save perhaps your own experience of having passed them.

A final remark: Goldsmith's literary fame brought him wealth and reputation, but his carelessness, intemperance and gambling habit brought him down and he died penniless, broken in health and mind, in 1774. Perhaps he would have benefited from familiarity with those professional competencies in our College's curriculum, which transcend knowledge, are not easily tested in exams, but will prove vital in you successfully meandering through your professional career, whether you play the flute or not.

Hugo de Waal MD, FRCPsych
Lead Clinician for North Norfolk
Head of School, Postgraduate School of Psychiatry,
East of England Deanery
College Tutor,
Norfolk and Waveney Psychiatric Training Scheme
Fellow, Higher Education Academy
August 2009

Preface

Having taken the first step towards successfully passing Paper II, your focus should be on finding answers to the most complex and difficult questions that you might expect in its exam. This book provides you with that and more, but first I would like to answer (for a change) some of the questions that trainees have often asked me.

WHEN IS THE RIGHT TIME TO SIT THE PAPER II EXAM?

In my opinion, the right time is your first opportunity to do so, as I think that the easiest way to become a Member is to focus on one exam at a time. However, if for any reason a person has to take Papers I and II together, that person should view the situation as a challenge befitting anyone who wants to pursue a career in psychiatry. Success comes with hard work.

HOW SHOULD I PREPARE FOR THE EXAM?

I have come across people who tend to rely on crash courses and then pass the exam on a wing and a prayer. Remember that the exam is a path, not just to becoming a Member, but also to having adequate knowledge to pursue a career in psychiatry. E is always equal to MC^2. If that were the focus, then reading for at least two hours a day during the specialty (core) training years 1 to 3 would give you a head start.

Once the exam day is getting nearer, intensive revision in a symbiotic relationship with a mould-forming kitchen sink would take you across the finish line in some style.

WHAT IS THE SYLLABUS FOR PAPER II?

The Department of Examinations, in their infinite wisdom, have never been content with what should constitute Paper II. At the time when specialty training was introduced, the syllabus was notably different to the syllabus that is current at the time of writing this book.

The current syllabus focuses on:

- general adult psychiatry
- epidemiology
- neuroscience
- psychopharmacology
- advanced psychological treatments.

The best way to keep track of this evolution is to visit www.rcpsych. ac.uk/training/examinations.aspx.

WILL THERE BE QUESTIONS OUTSIDE THE SYLLABUS?

Psychiatrists reside in the comfort zone of grey shades, and this applies to the exam, too! It is worth remembering that the idea behind the artificial division of the subject into three papers is to make learning a continuous activity that can be performed in manageable chunks. However, while setting the questions the line between what is psycho-pathology, what would be the psychopathological features of an illness that would affect prognosis, and what psychotherapy to choose for specific psychopathological features becomes a thin one. The College will make every effort to ensure that the exam adheres to the syllabus stringently, but that serves as guidance – not gospel. I would strongly recommend that trainees at least go through the psychopharmacology questions in *New MRCPsych Paper I Mock MCQ*!

DO I HAVE TO READ AND REMEMBER EVERYTHING UNDER THE SUN?

The important thing to do is to construct whatever you read into a question format. This should help you to recognise answers in multiple-choice questions, as you are unlikely to be questioned directly on what the incidence of schizophrenia is, but the question will present you with a narrative about a specific situation in which Mr Smith finds himself being the unfortunate last cousin of someone with a schizoid personality, and will then ask what his risk would be. Therefore thinking about facts and understanding their practical applications or theoretical underpinnings is what makes things easier during the exam.

Has this answered the question? Perhaps not. In simpler terms, recognising answers from sets of five options is all that you need to do. Now that comes with practice, which is why this book contains 650 such questions. The 3250 stems (which is what the choices are called) could be construed into individual facts, and questions could be formed from any one of them. The more you practise, the better the results will be.

WHAT SHALL I READ?

The important principle to remember is that the purpose of Papers 2 and 3 is to test for intensive understanding of a topic, not just superficial knowledge, and to test whether you keep abreast of emerging research evidence on the topics. I would advise you to read the *British Journal of Psychiatry*, *Advances in Psychiatric Treatments*, and some standard psychiatry textbooks, along with the National Institute for Health and Clinical Excellence (NICE) guidelines.

This is why this book contains questions that are referenced to the above-mentioned journals and the very latest textbooks – to give you a certain advantage over your peers who might have developed tunnel vision from restricting themselves to outdated information that has never been revised.

WILL THERE BE QUESTIONS THAT I CANNOT ANSWER HOWEVER HARD I TRY WHILE PREPARING?

The answer is yes. Still, these should be extremely few if you have worked hard, and should not be a cause for concern. In a similar vein, you will encounter some questions about which you might disagree with the examiners over the answers purely because of what the reference for an answer is, and also because psychiatry is rather a grey area.

And finally, best wishes with your studies. Luck can create an opportunity, but only hard work turns it into a success.

Vellingiri Badrakalimuthu
August 2009

About the author

Having completed the MBBS at Coimbatore Medical College, India, in 2002, Vellingiri trained in psychiatry at the Institute of Mental Health, Chennai, India. His first appointment in the UK was at the Maudsley Hospital, after which he took up a post as Senior House Officer on the Solent Rotation. He became a Member of the Royal College of Psychiatrists in 2007.

He has research publications to his credit and has been commissioned by Advances in Psychiatric Treatment and RCPsych-CPD Online for various projects. He has been shortlisted for the Advance Trainee of the Year Award (2009) by the Royal College of Psychiatrists. He is currently a registrar in Old Age Psychiatry and PBL tutor for CT1 and CT2 trainees. He is also studying for a Masters degree in Neuroscience at the Institute of Psychiatry, London.

About the references

JOURNALS

Advances in Psychiatric Treatment (2006, 2007, 2008 and 2009) (APT)
British Journal of Psychiatry (2006, 2007 and 2008) (BJP)

BOOKS

Hodges JR. *Cognitive Assessment for Clinicians*. Oxford: Oxford University Press; 2007. (CA)

Longstaff A. *Instant Notes in Neuroscience* (BIOS Instant Notes). Abingdon: Taylor & Francis; 2005. (N)

McGuffin P, Owen M, Gottesman I. *Psychiatric Genetics and Genomics*. Oxford: Oxford University Press; 2004. (PG)

Morgan G, Butler S. *Seminars in Basic Neurosciences*. 1993; www.rcpsych.ac.uk/pdf/semBasNeuro_prelims.pdf (SBN)

Patestas M, Gartner LP. *A Textbook of Neuroanatomy*. Oxford: Wiley-Blackwell; 2006. (TN)

Sadock B, Kaplan H, Sadock V. *Synopsis of Psychiatry. Behavioural Sciences/Clinical Psychiatry* (10 e). Philadelphia, PA: Lippincott Williams & Wilkins; 2007. (KS)

Scott AIF. *The ECT Handbook (2e): The Third Report of the Royal College of Psychiatrists' Special Committee on ECT*. London: Royal College of Psychiatrists; 2004. (ECT)

WEBSITES

www.nice.org.uk
www.rcpsych.ac.uk

To Hugo and Daphne

And still they gazed, and still the wonder grew.
That one small head could carry all he knew.

The Deserted Village
Oliver Goldsmith (1728–1774)

Paper 1

1. With regard to premenstrual syndrome, all of the following statements are true except:

   a. It is a research diagnosis in DSM-IV

   b. Symptoms occur in the luteal phase

   c. Symptoms remit for at least 1 week in the follicular phase

   d. The diagnosis is less stable over 48 months

   e. To be of clinical significance the symptoms should be of at least moderate intensity and cause severe functional impairment (APT 2007)

2. Which of the following statements about antidepressant discontinuation is true?

   a. Discontinuation symptoms are dependent on the underlying psychiatric disorder

   b. Discontinuation symptoms are not associated with mirtazapine

   c. It was first reported following the discontinuation of amitryptyline

   d. The mean duration of discontinuation syndrome is 2 weeks

   e. The onset of symptoms more than 1 week after discontinuation is unusual (APT 2007)

3. Regarding the treatment of mania, the following statements are all true except:

   a. Antipsychotics are the most commonly used drugs for patients hospitalised with mania

   b. Blockade of α_1 and H_1 receptors is hypothesised to contribute to the antimanic property of antipsychotics

   c. The NNT for olanzapine in the treatment of mania is 4

   d. Olanzapine acts faster in patients with non-psychotic mania than does valproate

   e. Olanzapine treatment predisposes to depression more than treatment with haloperidol during a phase of mania (APT 2008)

4. Which of the following statements about dangerous and severe personality disorder is true?

   a. According to the Department of Health definition, the risk presented should be functionally linked to personality disorder

   b. An admission to the DSPD unit requires one or more DSM-IV personality-disorder diagnoses

   c. Antisocial personality disorder is the second most common diagnosis among juvenile prisoners

   d. The minimum assessment required for admission to the DSPD unit does not require assessment on the International Personality Disorders Questionnaire

   e. Risk Matrix 2000 focuses on non-sexual offending (APT 2007)

5. Regarding the behavioural activation approach for depression, all of the following statements are true except:

   a. Behavioural activation is not about scheduling satisfying or pleasant events

   b. Behavioural activation uses the functional analysis of cognitive processes that involve avoidance

   c. Developmental formulation in behavioural activation shifts the emphasis away from its social context

   d. There is no significant difference between activity scheduling and activity scheduling with cognitive challenges

   e. There is no significant difference in 2-year outcomes between activity scheduling and activity scheduling with cognitive challenges to core beliefs and assumptions (APT 2008)

6. Which of the following statements is true regarding behavioural activation for depression?

   a. Goals should always include returning to normal work as soon as possible

   b. Learning theory is an alternative model to that of behavioural activation

   c. The number of sessions for treating depression is between 8 and 12

   d. Secondary coping behaviours are targeted when the individual is aware of precipitating factors

   e. The Valued Living Questionnaire offers prompts for values for the patient to decide on a Likert scale (APT 2008)

7. All of the following are approaches complementary to behavioural activation except:

    a. Acceptance and commitment therapy

    b. Compassionate mind training

    c. Family therapy

    d. Exercise and healthy eating

    e. Existential therapy (APT 2008)

8. Which of these statements about the epidemiology of paranoia is true?

    a. Delusions of reference are the second most common type of delusions

    b. Less than 1% of the non-clinical population have delusions of a level of severity comparable to that of clinical psychosis

    c. Odder, less plausible paranoid thoughts build on commoner, more plausible ones

    d. Persecutory delusions are found in post-traumatic stress disorder but not in epilepsy

    e. The rate of delusional beliefs in the general population is greater than that of psychosis (APT 2006)

9. Which of the following statements about the cognitive behaviour analysis system of psychotherapy (CBASP) is true?

    a. An interpersonal discrimination exercise is a conclusion that a patient draws with the assistance of the therapist about a significant other in the patient's life

    b. It was developed as a treatment for acute reactive depression

    c. Its key mechanism of change includes disciplined social involvement

    d. It uses its main therapy technique of situational analysis to ameliorate psychopathology during treatment sessions

    e. Its theoretical premise is that arrested maturational development is the aetiological basis of depression (APT 2007)

10. In CBASP, the therapist's personal involvement in the patient's problems to demonstrate for the patient that behaviour has consequences is part of which of the following?

    a. Contingent personal responsivity

    b. Disciplined personal involvement

    c. Hot spot

    d. Interpersonal discriminatory exercise

    e. 'Significant other' history (APT 2007)

11. Which of the following statements about CBASP is true?

    a. Contingent personal responsivity provides an opportunity to direct the patient's attention to the impact of the therapist's behaviour on the patient

    b. The Coping Survey Questionnaire is a type of Likert scale

    c. One way of analysing stimulus value is by using the Impact Message Inventory

    d. Situational analysis has three stages

    e. There is no significant difference between CBASP combined with drug therapy and drug therapy alone (APT 2007)

12. Which of the following statements about conversion disorder is true?

    a. According to DSM-IV criteria, conversion disorder is characterised by the involvement of psychological factors

    b. DSM-IV categorises conversion disorder and somatoform disorders separately

    c. Symptoms are common in children aged younger than 8 years

    d. Symptoms are most common in young males

    e. Around 10% of the patients admitted to general medical services have had conversion symptoms at some time in their life (APT 2009)

13. The Zurich criteria for hypomania include all of the following except:

   a. The absence of a past history of mania

   b. At least 3 of the 7 symptoms of hypomania according to DSM-IV

   c. Euphoria, irritability or over-activity

   d. Experience of negative consequences of hypomanic periods

   e. Hypomanic symptoms with a duration of at least 1 day (APT 2006)

14. Indicators of bipolarity in apparently unipolar depression include all of the following except:

   a. Antidepressant-induced mania or hypomania

   b. Early onset of depression

   c. Multiple family members with major depression

   d. Postpartum illness

   e. Psychotic features after the age of 35 years (APT 2006)

15. Regarding the use of IQ tests in the diagnosis of early schizophrenia, all of the following statements are true except:

   a. The average decline in IQ in samples with first-episode illness is generally less than that in groups with chronic schizophrenia

   b. In cases of suspected schizophrenia, a decline of 15 or more points indicates the presence of the disease

   c. National Adult Reading Test (NART) underestimates IQ decline in patients with schizophrenia

   d. People with schizophrenia on average have a lower IQ than the general population

   e. People with schizophrenia on average have a lower IQ than patients with bipolar disorder (APT 2008)

16. The therapeutic aims of long-term supportive psychotherapy in psychosis include all of the following except:

    a. Establishing a therapeutic alliance

    b. Holding and containing

    c. Promoting awareness of transference issues

    d. Promoting stability

    e. Providing rehabilitation pathways (APT 2008)

17. Which of the following is the therapeutic technique of long-term supportive psychotherapy?

    a. Cognitive reattribution

    b. Counselling

    c. Dynamic formulation

    d. Environmental interventions

    e. Relaxation training (APT 2008)

18. Which of the following statements about narcolepsy is true?

    a. Automatic behaviour is rare in patients with narcolepsy

    b. High concentrations of orexin A have been found in the CSF of patients with narcolepsy

    c. Overnight polysomnography reveals the presence of sleep-onset REM

    d. The prevalence of narcolepsy in the general population is 2.5%

    e. Sleep paralysis is seen in 75% of patients with narcolepsy (APT 2006)

19. Which of the following statements about sleep disorders is true?

    a. All episodes of behavioural disorder are associated with atonia in REM sleep disorder

    b. Clonazepam is contraindicated in patients with poor sleep in Guillain–Barré syndrome

    c. Episodes of behavioural disorder occur during the first third of sleep

    d. Individuals with non-REM sleep disorder act out their dreams

    e. Methylphenidate worsens cataleptic attacks (APT 2006)

20. All of the following statements about paranoid personality disorder are true except:

    a. Comorbidity with other personality disorders reaches up to 50%

    b. High levels of delinquency in teenagers have been associated with paranoid features

    c. Its prevalence in community samples is 1.3%

    d. Its prevalence among psychiatric outpatients is up to 10%

    e. Around 10% of people with paranoid personality disorder suffer from panic disorder (APT 2009)

21. With regard to the psychological processes in paranoid personality disorder, all of the following statements are true except:

    a. Attributional bias is a defence against low self-esteem

    b. Low levels of rumination are associated with aggression

    c. Paranoid thinking is associated with externalising personal attributional bias

    d. Paranoid thinking is associated with deficits in theory of mind

    e. Reciprocal determinism is a characteristic feature of the disorder (APT 2009)

22. All of the following are elements of the psychoanalytic theory of depression except:

    a. Ambivalence predisposes people to depression after object loss

    b. An excessively severe ego influences chronicity of depression

    c. Early feeding and affective bonding experiences are of particular importance in vulnerability to depression

    d. Somatic symptoms of depression arise from inhibited feelings of arousal

    e. The triangle of conflict includes feelings of anxiety and defence (APT 2009)

23. All of the following statements about spirituality are true except:

    a. Mental health professionals' attitudes towards spiritual care tend to be negative

    b. One of the areas of questioning recommended in the *Spirituality and Mental Health* leaflet from the Royal College of Psychiatrists is in regard to remedies

    c. Opinion polls indicate that although there has been a decline in religious beliefs, spirituality remains strong

    d. Psychiatric patients associate outcomes involving improved capacity for problem solving with spiritual care

    e. Within the literature, 20% of the studies identify spiritual or religious beliefs as being beneficial (APT 2007)

24. Which of the following statements about steroids is true?

    a. Anabolic steroids are prescription-only drugs

    b. Anabolic steroids are controlled drugs under class D

    c. Their circulating level of testosterone is typically 5% of that in males

    d. In a survey of college students in the UK, current steroid use or use during the previous year was 5%

    e. Around 10% of GPs treat patients who have engaged in steroid misuse (APT 2006)

25. Which of the following statements about the characteristics of steroids is true?

    a. Oxymetholone causes little liver toxicity

    b. Methenolone acetate causes severe water retention

    c. Nandrolone causes dose-dependent hypertension

    d. Stanozolol is injectable

    e. Testosterone enantate is long acting (APT 2006)

26. Which of the following matches is accurate with regard to drugs taken along with anabolic steroids?

    a. Clenbuterol – worsens asthma

    b. Cytomel – synthetic T_3

    c. Human growth hormone – high risk of hypoglycaemia

    d. Insulin-like growth factor – cardiomegaly

    e. Tamoxifen – oestrogen agonist (APT 2006)

27. All of the following statements about steroids and mental illness are true except:

    a. Depression is associated with withdrawing from steroids

    b. During steroid use, people score lower on schizoid personality traits

    c. The risk of developing psychotic symptoms may be related to high-dose testosterone

    d. Self-reported aggression may be the only sign of steroid misuse

    e. Steroid users have been shown to have a higher prevalence of cluster B personality traits (APT 2006)

28. Which of the following statements about the NICE guidelines for bipolar disorder is true?

    a. The annual cost of bipolar disorder in the UK is around £20 million

    b. Carbamazepine should not be used for the treatment of acute mania

    c. Paroxetine is the drug of choice for treating severe depression in pregnant women with bipolar disorder

    d. The incidence of bipolar disorder decreases from mid to late life

    e. The use of the Mood Disorder Questionnaire is advisable (www.nice.org.uk)

29. All of the following are NICE recommendations for the use of antidepressants in bipolar disorder except:

a. Anyone under the age of 30 years should be reviewed within 1 week for suicidal ideation

b. If the patient does not respond to three adequate trials of antidepressants, you should consider referral to a clinician with special interest

c. Lamotrigine can be used routinely to treat depressive episodes in bipolar type 1 disorder

d. Venlafaxine is less associated with discontinuation symptoms than are SSRIs

e. When the symptoms have been less severe for at least 8 weeks, the discontinuing of antidepressants should be considered (www.nice.org.uk)

30. Which of the following statements about the epidemiology of schizophrenia is true?

a. Around 80% of people with schizophrenia have persistent problems with social functioning

b. Around 60% of patients with schizophrenia are likely to relapse within 5 years of a treated first episode

c. The best predictor of a long-term prognosis is poor functioning in the first 2 years post diagnosis

d. Mortality among people with schizophrenia is 30% higher than that of the general population

e. Young women from diverse ethnic backgrounds are at a higher risk of suicide (KS)

31. Which of the following statements about schizophrenia patients' physical health is true?

   a. GPs are better than psychiatrists at recognising and treating physical health-related problems in people with schizophrenia

   b. GPs are as likely to screen individuals with schizophrenia for cardiovascular risk as they are to screen those with asthma

   c. Group intervention for smoking cessation has no significant impact on morbidity

   d. Patients with schizophrenia are less likely to attend screening for cardiovascular disorders than other people

   e. People with schizophrenia apparently do not have raised rates of lung cancer (www.nice.org.uk)

32. Which of the following statements about the management of schizophrenia is true?

   a. Around 10% of schizophrenia patients receiving first-generation antipsychotics develop tardive dyskinesia

   b. Fewer than 10% of service users are managed solely in primary care

   c. Raised serum prolactin levels from antipsychotics lead to reduced bone density

   d. Services for schizophrenia account for 40% of NHS spending on mental health

   e. Up to 25% of schizophrenia patients have a poor response to conventional antipsychotics (www.nice.org.uk)

33. Which of the following cranial nerves leaves the brainstem through the middle cerebellar peduncle?

   a. V

   b. VI

   c. VII

   d. VIII

   e. IX (TN)

34. The cranial nerve that arises between pyramids and olives is:

a. VIII

b. IX

c. X

d. XI

e. XII (TN)

35. The descending tract of the trigeminal nerve forms:

a. The fasciculus cuneatus

b. The fasciculus gracilis

c. The tuberculum cinereum

d. The tuberculum gracilis

e. The tuberculum cuneatus (TN)

36. Which of the following does the trigeminal ganglion occupy?

a. The diaphragm sella

b. The falx cerebri

c. The falx cerebelli

d. Meckel's cave

e. The tentorium cerebella (TN)

37. All of the following are correct with regard to the composition of cerebrospinal fluid except:

a. Calcium concentration is 1.0–1.4 mmol/L

b. Magnesium concentration is 0.8–1.3 mmol/L

c. pH is 7.3

d. Potassium concentration is 2.0–2.8 mmol/L

e. Protein – almost none (TN)

38. All of the following statements about the corticospinal tract are true except:

   a. Fibres terminating in the ventral motor horn of the spinal cord are involved in muscle contraction

   b. Fibres that do not decussate form the anterior corticospinal tract

   c. It passes through the posterior limb of the internal capsule near its genu

   d. It passes through the posterior half of the posterior limb of the internal capsule

   e. It passes through the upper third of the crux cerebri (TN)

39. Which of the following statements about the corticobulbar tract is correct?

   a. The corticonuclear tract descends posterior to the corticospinal tract

   b. The corticonuclear tract projects fibres bilaterally to the lower motor neuron of the facial nucleus that innervates muscles in the lower half of the face

   c. Its fibres terminate not only in target cranial nerve motor nuclei but also in the sensory relay nuclei

   d. The inferior colliculus relays corticonuclear fibres

   e. The lower motor neuron that innervates the genioglossus muscle receives bilateral corticonuclear projections (TN)

40. Mr Bainbridge presents with an inability to coordinate hand movements bilaterally, with no evidence of paralysis. At what level is his lesion?

   a. Corticospinal tract at the level of corona radiata

   b. Corticospinal tract at the level of crus cerebri

   c. Premotor cortex

   d. Primary motor cortex

   e. Supplementary motor area (TN)

41. Neostriatum is made of caudate and which of the following?

    a. Globus pallidus

    b. Nucleus accumbens

    c. Subthalamic nucleus

    d. Ventral pallidum

    e. Ventral tegmental area (TN)

42. Corticostriate fibres that terminate in the putamen use which of the following?

    a. Aspartate

    b. Dopamine

    c. Glycine

    d. Serotonin

    e. Arginine-vasopressin (TN)

43. Which of the following is the only cranial nerve to send central processes of some of its first-order neurons to synapse directly in the cerebellum?

    a. III

    b. V

    c. VII

    d. VIII

    e. XI (TN)

44. The carotid sinus reflex would be lost in a lesion involving which of the following?

    a. The inferior ganglion of glossopharyngeal nerve

    b. The jugular ganglion of vagus nerve

    c. The otic ganglion of glossopharyngeal nerve

    d. The superior ganglion of glossopharyngeal nerve

    e. The superior ganglion of vagus nerve (TN)

45. Which of the following is the nucleus involved in phonation?

    a. Ambiguus

    b. Dorsal motor nucleus of vagus

    c. Hypoglossal

    d. Solitarius

    e. Spinal nucleus of trigeminal (TN)

46. In which of the following are the cell bodies of rods and cones present?

    a. Ganglion cell layer

    b. Inner nuclear layer

    c. Outer nuclear layer

    d. Optic nerve fibre layer

    e. Rod and cone layer (TN)

47. Which of the following statements about the optic pathway is true?

    a. The axons of the optic nerve become myelinated once they pierce the lamina cribrosa

    b. The optic chiasma sends fibres to the hypothalamus

    c. The secondary visual cortex involves the middle temporal area

    d. The sublenticular portion of the geniculocalcarine tract goes up to the cuneate gyrus

    e. The first-order neurons are pseudounipolar (TN)

48. All of the following statements about the primary somatosensory cortex are true except:

a. The area within the central sulcus receives input from muscle receptors

b. It includes the dorsal part of the paracentral lobule

c. The primary auditory cortex includes the transverse temporal gyri of Heschl

d. The primary visual cortex receives input from the macula of retina in its rostral portions

e. A solitary nucleus transmits taste sensation to the postcentral gyrus through the ventroposteromedial nucleus of the thalamus (TN)

49. All of the following statements about the cortex are true except:

a. Broca's area consists of supramarginal gyrus

b. The dorsolateral prefrontal cortex functions in working memory

c. The secondary auditory cortical areas are connected with Wernicke's area

d. The somaesthetic association area is located in the superior parietal lobule

e. Tertiary visual areas include the middle temporal area of the cortex (TN)

50. Mr Bainbridge presents with cortical blindness. This is due to an infarction involving which of the following?

a. The anterior cerebral artery

b. The anterior communicating artery

c. The basilar artery

d. The middle cerebral artery

e. The posterior communicating artery (TN)

51. Mr Bainbridge presents with a deviation of both his eyes to the right side. This is due to a lesion involving which of the following?

a. The left frontal eye field

b. The left primary visual area

c. The right frontal eye field

d. The right primary visual area

e. The right visual association area (TN)

52. Mr Bainbridge presents with difficulty in processing what he hears and formulating a response. However, he can comprehend what he hears, and his language expression is fluent. At which level is the lesion?

a. The arcuate fasciculus

b. Broca's area

c. The primary auditory cortex

d. The transcortical global

e. Wernicke's area (TN)

53. Which of the following statements about pain sensation is true?

a. The activation of large myelinated mechanoreceptor afferents can reduce some forms of pain

b. The anterior nucleus of the hypothalamus is involved in the pathways for discriminating aspects of somaesthesia

c. Burning sensations are thought to be carried by small myelinated Aδ fibres

d. The electrical stimulation of the raphe nucleus produces profound hyperaesthesia

e. The spinal-cord neurons that relay pain sensation are located in the deep laminae of the dorsal grey matter (SBN)

54. Which of the following statements is true?

a. Clasp knife reflex is mediated by interneurons which are connected to 1a fibres

b. The GABA-secreting interneurons of basal ganglia are co-localised with somatostatin

c. Group 1b afferent axons have excitatory connections with the motor neurons that cause muscle to contract

d. The intrinsic neurons of the cerebellum exclude excitatory granule cells

e. The motor neurons in the spinal cord form the final common path for all motor activity (SBN)

55. Which of the following statements about visual pathways is true?

a. Layers 1, 4 and 6 of the lateral geniculate nucleus receive input from the ipsilateral temporal retina

b. A small portion of nasal hemiretina that receives monocular vision is called a nasal crescent

c. The superior colliculus is responsible for directing each fovea to its target

d. A unilateral lesion of the frontal cortex results in the inability to direct a gaze laterally in either direction

e. The vestibular nuclei send information to the cranial nuclei of the second nerve (SBN)

56. Which of the following statements about vestibular reflexes is incorrect?

   a. Compensatory eye movement has two phases

   b. Defects associated with the fast phase are related to reticular formation

   c. Four vestibular nuclei are located in the medulla

   d. The inferior vestibular nucleus plays the key role in reflex control of head position

   e. The lateral vestibular nucleus receives inhibitory input from the cerebellum (SBN)

57. Which of the following statements about reticular formation is true?

   a. Colliculi are involved in orienting the head towards the direction of startle stimuli

   b. EEG changes are independent of the effects of the thalamic nuclei on the cerebral cortex

   c. The startle response is independent of reticular formation

   d. Stimulation of the nucleus raphe magnus produces hyperaesthesia

   e. Stimulation of the reticular formation leads to the extinction of aversive behaviour (SBN)

58. Which of the following forms of apraxia accompanies Broca's aphasia?

   a. Conceptual

   b. Dressing

   c. Ideomotor

   d. Limb kinetic

   e. Oral (CA)

59. Mr Bainbridge presents with an inability to carry out motor tasks to command, but performs the same tasks spontaneously. At which of the following is the lesion?

a. The basal ganglion

b. The inferior frontal region

c. The left frontotemporal area

d. The left parietal lobe

e. The right posterior parietal area (CA)

60. Mr Bainbridge presents with an inability to name or describe visually presented items. Which of the following does the lesion involve?

a. The bilateral posterior occipitoparietal region

b. The bilateral temporoparietal region

c. The left anterior temporal lobe

d. The left medial occipital region

e. The occipitotemporal area (CA)

61. All of the following statements about Balint's syndrome are true except:

a. It involves a lesion of angular gyrus

b. There is an inability to reach for visual targets

c. There is an inability to point at visual targets

d. Simultagnosia is a feature

e. Symptoms include an inability to direct voluntary eye movements to visual targets (CA)

62. Mr Bainbridge presents with impairment in retrieval of colour information. This is which of the following?

a. Achromatopsia

b. Apperceptive visual agnosia

c. Colour agnosia

d. Prosopagnosia

e. Simultagnosia (CA)

63. Which of the following do phakomatoses include?

a. Arteriovenous malformations

b. Fragile X syndrome

c. Heterotopia of grey matter

d. Schizencephaly

e. Tuberous sclerosis (SBN)

64. Based on a presentation of hypertelorism, high arched palate, absent patellae, congenital heart disease and agenesis of corpus callosum, which of the following is the correct chromosomal abnormality?

a. 5p deletion

b. 8 mosaic

c. 9p trisomy

d. 22 trisomy

e. XXY (SBN)

65. Based on a presentation of infantile hypotonia, learning disability, short stature, small hands and feet, hypoplastic genitalia, hyperphagia and obesity, which of the following is the correct chromosomal abnormality?

    a. 5p deletion

    b. 15 deletion

    c. 18p deletion

    d. 21 trisomy

    e. XO (SBN)

66. Which of the following is the atresia of foramen of Luschka and Magendie associated with hydrocephalus?

    a. An Arnold–Chiari malformation

    b. An Aicardi malformation

    c. A Dandy–Walker malformation

    d. Bourneville's disease

    e. Von Hippel–Lindau disease (SBN)

67. In which of the following are tuber-like astrocytic lesions seen?

    a. Bourneville's disease

    b. The De Lange malformation

    c. Encephalofacial angiomatosis

    d. Sturge–Weber syndrome

    e. Von Recklinghausen's syndrome (SBN)

68. Which of the following is the commonest form of primitive neuroectodermal tumour?

a. Astrocytoma

b. Ependymoma

c. Oligodendroglioma

d. Medulloblastoma

e. Microglioma (SBN)

69. All of the following statements about cranial tumours are true except:

a. Anterior falx meningiomas may present with the frontal lobe syndrome

b. Limbic encephalitis can be a non-metastatic complication of systemic malignant disease

c. Malignant tumours are more common in the anterior pituitary than in the posterior pituitary

d. Meningiomas commonly originate from the arachnoid cells of leptomeninges

e. Metastases are usually from carcinomas of the lung (SBN)

70. Which of the following elements is associated with cerebellar damage, damage to primary sensory areas, and neurasthenic syndrome?

a. Aluminium

b. Copper

c. Chlorine

d. Lead

e. Mercury (SBN)

71. Which of the following is damaged by MPTP?

    a. Nucleus basalis of Meynert

    b. Locus coeruleus

    c. Mamillary body

    d. Raphe nucleus

    e. Substantia nigra (SBN)

72. Deficiency of which of these vitamins causes subacute combined degeneration of the spinal cord?

    a. Cyanocobalamin

    b. Folate

    c. Niacin

    d. Riboflavin

    e. Thiamine (SBN)

73. All of the following statements about neuropeptide Y(NPY) are true except:

    a. It is not synthesised in the cell bodies of the paraventricular nucleus

    b. It controls luteinising hormones, releasing the hormone in the absence of oestrogen priming

    c. It controls the thyrotropin-releasing hormone

    d. It is co-localised with catecholamines in neurons that originate from the brainstem

    e. It is not co-localised with catecholamines in neurons that originate from the arcuate nucleus (SBN)

74. All of the following stimulate feeding except:

   a. Galanin

   b. Growth-hormone-releasing factor

   c. Opioids

   d. Neuropeptide Y

   e. Neurotensin (SBN)

75. Which of the following inhibits feeding?

   a. Cholecystokinin

   b. Galanin

   c. Growth-hormone-releasing factor

   d. Neuropeptide Y

   e. Noradrenaline through α_2-receptors (SBN)

76. All of the following stimulate the release of arginine vasopressin except:

   a. Atrial peptides

   b. Decreased plasma osmolality

   c. Hypovolaemia

   d. Nausea

   e. Stress (SBN)

77. Which of the following is the hypothalamic nucleus involved in the control of gonadotrophin-releasing hormone?

   a. The arcuate nucleus

   b. The paraventricular nucleus

   c. The periventricular nucleus

   d. The preoptic area

   e. The supraoptic nucleus (SBN)

78. All of the following statements about the genetics of autism are true except:

    a. The candidate gene for autism is the 5HT transporter gene

    b. The concordance rate among MZ twins has ranged from 36% to 90%

    c. A LOD score of 2.53 is reported in a region on chromosome 7q

    d. The relative increased risk to siblings of those with classic autism is between 10 and 20

    e. Tuberous sclerosis occurs in less than 5% of those with autism (PG)

79. Which of the following is true with regard to the genetics of childhood schizophrenia?

    a. An association with abnormality of D_3 receptor locus has been reported for adult- but not childhood-onset schizophrenia

    b. The concordance rate among MZ twins is lower than that of adult-onset schizophrenia

    c. Chromosome 1p22 has been implicated

    d. The rate of deletion of chromosome 22q11 is lower than that seen in adult schizophrenia

    e. The rate of non-affective psychosis among relatives of childhood schizophrenics with premorbid speech and language impairment is lower than that in the adult population with schizophrenia (PG)

80. Which of the following statements about the genetics of ADHD is true?

a. The DAT2 gene has been implicated in ADHD

b. The DRD4 7 allele confers susceptibility with an estimated odds ratio of between 2.5 and 3.0

c. Family studies have shown that ADHD and conduct disorders are co-transmitted among families

d. The relative risk of ADHD among first-degree relatives is greater among probands with ADHD that persists into adult life than among probands with ADHD that is comorbid with conduct disorder

e. First-degree relatives have a relative risk of between 2 and 3 (PG)

81. All of the following statements about the genetics of personality disorders are true except:

a. An increased rate of schizophrenia has been found among first-degree relatives of probands with schizotypal disorder

b. An increased rate of schizotypal personality disorder has been found among the relatives of patients with schizophrenia

c. Studies have generally reported negative results for borderline personality disorder among first-degree relatives of patients with depression

d. Studies have reported a higher rate of Briquet syndrome among the female relatives of males with antisocial personality disorder

e. Studies have reported that lying has more genetic heritability than truancy, which shows a stronger influence from shared environmental effects (PG)

82. Which of the following statements about the genetics of bipolar disorder is true?

a. Bipolar disorder type 2 is found with less frequency in the families of bipolar type 1 probands than in the general population

b. The MZ concordance for narrowly defined bipolar disorder is 30%

c. The number of affected relatives is a marker for familial disorder, but a vulnerability to puerperal triggering of episodes is not

d. Pre-pubertal depression has a distinct genetic aetiology

e. There is an estimated risk of 7% for bipolar disorder type 1 among first-degree relatives of cases with the same disorder (PG)

83. All of the following statements about adrenergic receptors are true except:

a. β_2-receptors are presynaptic inhibitory autoreceptors

b. cAMP is reduced by α_2-receptors

c. cAMP-mediated phosphorylation of N-type Ca^{2+} channels reduces noradrenaline release

d. GO second messenger, coupled to $\alpha1$-receptor, reduces gK

e. Gs is the second messenger system involved in β-receptors (N)

84. Which of the following is true with regard to serotonin?

a. Choroid plexus lacks serotonergic innervation

b. Ecstasy increases the release of serotonin

c. The oxidative decarboxylation of serotonin by MAO yields 5-HIAA

d. Serotonergic cells are important for learning about aversive situations

e. Serotonin synthesis is independent of the firing frequency of neurons (N)

85. At which of the following serotonin receptors is ketanserin an antagonist?

    a. 1a

    b. 1b

    c. 2a

    d. 2b

    e. 3 (N)

86. Ondansetron increases IP$_3$ levels by acting at which of the following serotonergic receptor subtypes?

    a. 1a

    b. 2b

    c. 3

    d. 4

    e. 7^d (N)

87. Sumatriptan is an agonist at which of the following serotonergic receptors?

    a. 1b

    b. 1d

    c. 2a

    d. 2b

    e. 3 (N)

88. Which of the following enzymes is used in the polymerase chain reaction?

    a. DNA trinucleotidase

    b. Restriction endonuclease

    c. Reverse transcriptase

    d. RNA polymerase

    e. Taq polymerase (PG)

89. A micro-array is called which of the following?

 a. A DNA chip

 b. A polymerase chain reaction

 c. A primer extension

 d. A restriction fragment length polymorphism

 e. A short tandem repeat polymorphism (PG)

90. By which of the following methods can mRNA be assayed?

 a. Central blotting

 b. Eastern blotting

 c. Northern blotting

 d. Southern blotting

 e. Western blotting (PG)

91. By which of the following methods can DNA be assayed?

 a. Central blotting

 b. Eastern blotting

 c. Northern blotting

 d. Southern blotting

 e. Western blotting (PG)

92. Which of the following is Mendel's law?

 a. Dependent assortment

 b. Incomplete penetrance

 c. Integration

 d. Segregation

 e. Variable expressivity (PG)

93. Which of the following genes has been implicated in determining precortical volume decline in people with schizophrenia?

    a. COMT

    b. DISC1

    c. Dysbindin

    d. Neuregulin

    e. PRODH (BJP 2006)

94. Which of the following genes has been implicated in learning and memory in the disease model of schizophrenia?

    a. COMT

    b. DISC1

    c. Dysbindin

    d. Neuregulin

    e. PRODH (BJP 2006)

95. Which of the following genes interacts with LIS1 to cause lissencephaly?

    a. COMT

    b. DISC1

    c. Dysbindin

    d. Neuregulin

    e. PRODH (BJP 2006)

96. Which of the following genes is associated with mitochondrial and microtubule function?

    a. COMT

    b. DISC1

    c. Dysbindin

    d. Neuregulin

    e. PRODH (BJP 2006)

97. All of the following statements about cognitive impairment in bipolar disorder are true except:

    a. Cognitive impairment in bipolar disorder remits during phases of euthymia

    b. Medium-term lithium treatment does not impair explicit memory

    c. The occurrence of psychotic symptoms is related to poor performance on cognitive tasks

    d. One predictor of a poor prognosis in bipolar type 2 disorder is poor performance on executive-function tasks

    e. Working memory is impaired in bipolar disorder (BJP 2006)

98. Which of the following statements about hysteria is true?

    a. Hoover's sign of paralysis has poor reliability for differentiating conversion from organic disorder

    b. La belle indifference is not a diagnostic criterion

    c. La belle indifference is an important discriminant between organic and conversion disorders

    d. La belle indifference is linked to left-hemisphere pathology

    e. The midline splitting of sensory loss has good reliability for distinguishing conversion disorder from organic disorder (BJP 2006)

99. Which of the following statements about insight and cognition is true?

    a. The analysis of different insight scales reveals a differential association with cognitive performance

    b. Impaired insight is not associated with the severity of the pathology

    c. Impaired insight is not associated with prefrontal dysfunction

    d. Impaired insight is significantly correlated with neurocognitive performance

    e. The relationship between IQ and insight is stronger than the relationship between insight and WCST scores (BJP 2006)

100. Which of the following statements about memory impairment in schizophrenia is true?

    a. A minority of community-based patients have memory deficits

    b. The Rivermead Behavioural Memory Test has 8 items

    c. A significant inverse correlation exists between age and memory scores

    d. A significant correlation exists between a positive scale of PANSS and memory scores

    e. A significant correlation exists between type of antipsychotic and memory scores (BJP 2006)

101. Which of the following statements about clozapine is true?

   a. Carbamazepine is safe, as it does not increase the possibility of neutropenia

   b. Clozapine must be stopped immediately if the white cell count falls below 5×10^9

   c. Clozapine must be stopped immediately if the neutrophil count falls below 3×10^9

   d. Infection can be a precipitant of neutropenia in patients who are challenged with clozapine

   e. Patients who develop neutropenia should not be rechallenged with clozapine (BJP 2006)

102. All of the following statements about panic disorder are true except:

   a. In acute-phase treatment, combined treatment is superior to antidepressant treatment

   b. Beyond its acute phase, combined treatment is superior to antidepressant treatment

   c. Beyond its acute phase, combined treatment is superior to psychotherapy

   d. The evidence for cognitive–behavioural therapy is most conclusive

   e. Pharmacotherapy is associated with significant relapse rates even when patients are maintained on adequate doses of antidepressants (BJP 2006)

103. An MRS study of patients with Alzheimer's disease found their inositol levels to be increased. In which of the following is this change seen?

   a. Frontal

   b. Insular

   c. Occipital

   d. Parietal

   e. Temporal (KS)

104. All of the following statements about fMRI are true except:

a. fMRI shows that the neural circuit for lexical categories involves the left anterior temporal lobe

b. fMRI shows that the area activated upon listening to speech is also activated during auditory hallucinations in people with schizophrenia

c. fMRI shows that patients with dyslexia show a failure to activate Wernicke's area

d. It gives specific information about neuronal metabolism

e. It works on the principle of detecting the levels of oxygenation in blood (KS)

105. All of the following statements about adult ADHD are true except:

a. About 65% of those with ADHD fulfil the criteria for partial remission at the age of 25 years

b. ADHD symptoms are continuously distributed throughout the population

c. ADHD symptoms show an age-dependent decline

d. Adults with ADHD respond to stimulants

e. Longitudinal studies show that ADHD and antisocial behaviour start simultaneously (BJP 2007)

106. All of the following statements about the treatment and outcomes of eating disorders among adolescents are true except:

a. High expressed emotion is associated with poor outcomes

b. Inpatient treatment predicts poor outcomes

c. Only about 50% of adolescents adhere to inpatient treatment

d. There is RCT evidence for family treatment for anorexia in adolescents

e. Those receiving lengthy inpatient treatment that results in their regaining normal weight continue to maintain their weight at 1-year follow-up (BJP 2007)

107. All of the following statements about depression and MI are true except:

    a. An ENRICHD study showed that the improvement in depression observed at 6 months following CBT was sustained at 30 months

    b. Post-MI depression is associated with a 2- to 2.5-fold increase in mortality

    c. Sertraline is a safe drug to use in post-MI patients

    d. The somatic symptoms of depression are associated with a poor prognosis in post-MI patients

    e. CBT has no effect on the risk of all-cause mortality in MI patients with depression (BJP 2007)

108. Which of the following is an agent that binds to the same receptor as an agonist for that receptor, but produces the opposite pharmacological effect?

    a. Antagonist

    b. Full agonist

    c. Inverse agonist

    d. Mixed agonist

    e. Partial agonist (KS)

109. Which of the following drugs is associated with weight loss?

    a. Bupropion

    b. Buspirone

    c. Lithium

    d. Sodium valproate

    e. Topiramate (KS)

110. Serious exfoliative dermatitis is seen with:

    a. Clonazepam

    b. Lamotrigine

    c. Phenytoin

    d. Sodium valproate

    e. Vigabatrin (KS)

111. Which of the following is an antipsychotic associated with high muscarinic blockade?

    a. Aripiprazole

    b. Olanzapine

    c. Risperidone

    d. Quetiapine

    e. Ziprasidone (KS)

112. Rabbit syndrome can be treated using:

    a. Buspirone

    b. Clonazepam

    c. Diphenhydramine

    d. Orphenadrine

    e. Propranolol (KS)

113. Which of the following statements about untreated psychosis is true?

    a. Its acute onset is associated with a substantially longer duration of untreated psychosis

    b. The duration of untreated psychosis lacks correlation with mid-term outcomes

    c. Family help-seeking is associated with a shorter duration of the untreated illness

    d. Unemployment is not related to the duration of untreated psychosis

    e. Unlike psychosis, the duration of untreated illness has no effect on the prognosis for anxiety disorders (BJP 2006)

114. All of the following statements about vagus stimulation are true except:

    a. The acute response to vagus stimulation in resistant depression is notably low

    b. It has been found to be effective in the treatment of resistant epilepsy

    c. The leads from the device are connected to the thoracic vagus

    d. The procedure involves the subcutaneous implantation of a pacemaker-like device

    e. Vocal cord palsy has been reported to be an adverse effect of the procedure (BJP 2006)

115. Which of the following statements about violence and psychiatric comorbidity is true?

    a. An increased risk of violence in youth is dependent on psychiatric comorbidity

    b. A large reduction in exposure to the risk factor of hazardous drinking at the individual level is associated with a large overall impact on a population's behaviour with regard to drinking

    c. People with psychotic illness pose a greater threat to random members of the public than to people they know

    d. The public health impact of violence from schizophrenia is lower than that from substance use

    e. Low self-esteem is associated with the risk of violence by men against their partners, but somatic complaints are not (BJP 2006)

116. All of the following statements about velocardio-facial syndrome (VCF) and facial-expression processing are true except:

    a. Facial processing networks involve occipital gyri providing input to the superior temporal region

    b. VCF is associated with chromosome 22q11 deletion

    c. People with VCF perform less well on space-perception tasks than on object-perception tasks

    d. People with VCF show less activation of their right insula in facial processing

    e. People with VCF show more activation of their bilateral occipital lobes in early facial processing (BJP 2006)

117. Which of the following statements about psychotherapy is true?

    a. Antidepressant therapy is as effective as combined therapy in the treatment of panic disorder without agoraphobia

    b. Brief, dynamic psychotherapy is more effective than CBT for avoidant personality disorder

    c. Music therapy significantly improves the general symptoms of schizophrenia

    d. Younger patients with first- and second-episode psychosis respond better to counselling than to CBT

    e. Younger patients with first- and second-episode psychosis show greater insight after counselling than after CBT (BJP 2006)

118. All of the following are good prognostic factors for brief psychotic disorder except:

    a. Affective symptoms

    b. Confusion during onset

    c. Insidious onset

    d. Little affective blunting

    e. Severe precipitating stressor (KS)

119. Which of the following statements about brief psychotic disorders is true?

    a. DSM-IV-TR describes four subtypes

    b. Less than half of the patients with these disorders display schizophrenia or mood disorder at long-term follow-up

    c. A longer duration of symptoms is associated with a good prognosis

    d. They are more common in older patients

    e. Psychodynamic formulations suggest that such psychotic symptoms develop as defences against prohibited fantasies (KS)

120. Which of the following is an anger syndrome associated with insomnia, fatigue, fear of impending death, dysphoric affect, indigestion, and the feeling of a mass in the epigastrium?

a. Brain fag

b. Dhat

c. Hwa-byung

d. Koro

e. Locura (KS)

121. Which of the following statements about psychodynamic factors in depression is true?

a. According to Melanie Klein, depression is an expression of anger towards hated people

b. According to self-psychological theory, when the developing needs of the self are unmet, a massive loss of self-esteem results

c. Damaged early attachment predisposes people to childhood depression

d. Disturbances in the genital phase predispose people to subsequent vulnerability to depression

e. The projection of departed objects is a defence mechanism for dealing with distress resulting from object loss (KS)

122. Beliefs about oneself, the world and the future are referred to as:

a. Cognitive distortion

b. The cognitive triad

c. Learned helplessness

d. Schema

e. Psychodynamic hierarchies (KS)

123. The forming of conclusions based on too little and too narrow experience is referred to as:

    a. Arbitrary inference

    b. Magnification and minimisation

    c. Oversimplification

    d. Personalisation

    e. Specific abstraction (KS)

124. The tendency to put experiences into all-or-nothing categories is referred to as:

    a. Absolutist thinking

    b. Arbitrary inference

    c. Oversimplification

    d. Personalisation

    e. Specific abstraction (KS)

125. All of the following statements about the course of major depressive disorder are true except:

    a. Around 5–10% of patients with an initial diagnosis of depression develop a manic episode 6 to 10 years after initial diagnosis

    b. Late onset is associated with antisocial personality disorder

    c. A major depressive disorder is usually preceded by a premorbid personality disorder

    d. Over a 20-year period the mean number of episodes is between five and six

    e. Untreated episodes last for about 6 to 13 months (KS)

126. Which of the following is a selection criterion for time-limited psychotherapy?

    a. The ability to engage and disengage

    b. Low ego strength

    c. Being unsuitable for borderline personality disorder

    d. Being unsuitable for major depressive disorder

    e. The therapist being quickly able to identify a central issue (KS)

127. For which of the following is the use of projection and splitting as defence mechanisms specifically unsuitable?

    a. Brief focal psychotherapy

    b. Psychoanalytic psychotherapy

    c. Short-term anxiety-provoking psychotherapy

    d. Short-term dynamic psychotherapy

    e. Time-limited psychotherapy (KS)

128. Abreaction is used as a major group process in:

    a. Analytically oriented group therapy

    b. Behavioural group therapy

    c. Psychoanalysis of groups

    d. Supportive group therapy

    e. Transactional group therapy (KS)

129. In which of the following is socialisation outside the group always encouraged?

    a. Analytically oriented group therapy

    b. Behavioural group therapy

    c. Psychoanalysis of groups

    d. Supportive group therapy

    e. Transactional group therapy (KS)

130. Improving adaptation to the environment is a goal of:

    a. Analytically oriented group therapy

    b. Behavioural group therapy

    c. Psychoanalysis of groups

    d. Supportive group therapy

    e. Transactional group therapy (KS)

Paper 2

1. With regard to the epidemiology of premenstrual syndrome, which of the following statements is true?

   a. Its diagnosis is associated with smoking and higher educational levels

   b. Fewer than 10% of women with the syndrome miss work

   c. The lifetime rate for comorbid post-traumatic stress disorder is high

   d. Premenstrual dysphoric disorder has a prevalence of between 15% and 20%

   e. Women with this syndrome score as badly as those with dysthymia on the Parental Factor of the Social Adjustment Scale Self-Report (APT 2007)

2. All of the following statements about the symptoms of antidepressant discontinuation are true except:

   a. The discontinuation syndrome associated with tranylcypromine is more severe than that associated with other antidepressants

   b. Dizziness and nausea are the most common symptoms

   c. Dystonia has been observed with the discontinuation of fluoxetine

   d. Sensory abnormalities are specific to discontinuation of tricyclic antidepressants

   e. Brief bursts of disequilibrium symptoms are associated with primary discontinuation syndrome (APT 2007)

3. Which of the following statements about cannabis is true?

   a. Cannabis is the second most commonly used psychoactive drug

   b. Cannabis use is reaching a plateau phase in high-income countries

   c. Cannabis use causes more harm to public health than tobacco use

   d. Approximately one-third of UK adolescents use cannabis at least once

   e. One of the most effective ways to reduce cannabis use among young people is through school-based interventions (APT 2007)

4. All of the following statements about cannabis are true except:

   a. Between 20% and 70% of people with severe mental illness use cannabis

   b. Cannabis use is more common among people with severe mental illness than in the general population

   c. The tetrahydrocannabinol content of skunk has doubled in the last 10 years

   d. A dose-dependent relationship exists between cannabis use and psychosis

   e. Strong evidence exists that cannabis use at a young age is linked to the development of severe mental illness (APT 2008)

5. Cannabis use among severely mentally ill people is associated with all of the following except:

   a. Increased criminal activity

   b. Increased rates of suicide

   c. Longer admissions

   d. Poorer physical health

   e. Reduced polysubstance use (APT 2008)

6. With regard to the assessment tools for use with patients with cannabis misuse and psychosis, which of the following statements is true?

    a. The Addiction Severity Index does not include psychiatric problems

    b. Patients with schizotypal personality disorder report fewer unpleasant after-effects on the Cannabis Experiences Questionnaire

    c. The Psychiatric Research Interview for Substance and Mental Disorders takes less time to complete than scheduled interviews

    d. The Stages of Change Readiness and Treatment Eagerness Scale is a 15-item self-report measure

    e. The Substance Use Scale for Psychosis can be used to explore patients' reasons for using drugs (APT 2008)

7. Examining the evidence base of psychological therapies for cannabis use shows that all of the following statements are correct except:

    a. The DATOS-A showed significant improvement in the reduction of suicidal thoughts and hostility among 11- to 18-year-olds

    b. The DATOS-A shows the superiority of outpatient over inpatient programmes

    c. Motivational enhancement therapy reduces the use of cannabis among 16- to 20-year-olds

    d. Psychological intervention achieves sustained abstinence in 14–22% of its patients for the 12-month period following the interventions

    e. Psychological therapy with contingency management is associated with better outcomes than psychological therapy alone (APT 2008)

8. Which of the following statements about the neuropathology of conversion disorders is true?

   a. They involve the impairment of the non-dominant hemisphere only

   b. The impairment that they cause is restricted to sub-cortical functioning

   c. They are associated with PET evidence of high blood flow in the thalamus

   d. They involve a reduction in the activity of the orbitofrontal cortex

   e. Sub-cortical asymmetry resolves with treatment (APT 2006)

9. Mr Jones suffers from conversion disorder and has been referred to your services by a neurologist. All of the following statements are true except:

   a. Acute conversion symptoms may undergo spontaneous resolution with the use of explanation and suggestion

   b. A high level of psychiatric comorbidity is associated with conversion disorder

   c. RCT showed that the addition of hypnotherapy to a comprehensive hospital treatment programme did not have any additional effect on treatment outcomes

   d. The recovery phase of chronic conversion disorder may reveal an underlying psychosis

   e. There is a lack of evidence to suggest that patients with conversion disorder have above-average hypnosibility (APT 2006)

10. Which of the following statements about race, ethnicity, culture and psychotherapy is true?

a. All therapists should avoid shared projection and acculturation gaps

b. Ethnicity is a social construct that defines a group by its members' race, colour, nationality, ethnicity or national origins

c. Psychotherapists need to be proficient in culture-bound mythology

d. Race-based transference uses splitting but not projection as a defence mechanism

e. Empirical evidence suggests that ethnic matching improves outcomes in therapy (APT 2007)

11. Which of the following statements about the genetic and developmental aspects of schizophrenia is true?

a. Clinical symptoms in first-degree relatives of patients with schizophrenia are restricted to positive ones

b. Most people with schizophrenia have an onset in late adolescence or adulthood

c. Older children without thought disorders tend to score higher on thought-disorder indices than younger children

d. Schizotaxia is apparent in 10% of first-degree relatives of people with schizophrenia

e. An underlying vulnerability to disorders in the schizophrenia spectrum begins to manifest with positive symptoms (APT 2007)

12. All of the following statements about the prodrome of schizophrenia are true except:

    a. An analysis of the school reports of patients with schizophrenia showed differences in their childhood social behaviour compared with that of the general population

    b. Children at high genetic risk of schizophrenia exhibit deficits in working memory

    c. Children who later develop schizophrenia present with lower premorbid IQ

    d. Deficits in sustained attention are seen in asymptomatic biological relatives of patients with schizophrenia

    e. Studies of children who have mothers with schizophrenia suggest that early development is normal but not sustained (APT 2007)

13. The client factors that are suitable for long-term psychodynamic psychotherapy include all of the following except:

    a. Treatment-resistant psychosis

    b. The presence of previous severe disruption to personality development

    c. The presence of a lack of consistent problem focus

    d. The presence of unhelpful team reactions that have become obstacles to offering care

    e. Willingness to take responsibility for addressing problems (APT 2008)

14. The percentage of people who show a steady progression of disability from multiple sclerosis is:

    a. 1–4%

    b. 5–10%

    c. 11–15%

    d. 16–20%

    e. 21–25% (APT 2006)

15. The lifetime risk of multiple sclerosis in the UK is:

    a. 1 in 8 000 000

    b. 1 in 800 000

    c. 1 in 80 000

    d. 1 in 8000

    e. 1 in 800 (APT 2006)

16. What is the prevalence of depression among patients with multiple sclerosis as opposed to the rest of the population?

    a. Twofold higher

    b. Threefold higher

    c. Fivefold higher

    d. Tenfold higher

    e. Twenty-fold higher (APT 2006)

17. The risk factors for suicide among patients with multiple sclerosis include all of the following except:

    a. Female gender

    b. Past history of depression

    c. Social isolation

    d. Substance misuse

    e. Young age of onset (APT 2006)

18. All of the following statements about the practice of psycho-dynamic psychotherapy are true except:

   a. A 5-year follow-up study showed that psychodynamic psychotherapy reduced recovery time

   b. An effect size of 0.76 has been found for all forms of psychological therapy in the treatment of non-psychotic disorders

   c. An effect size of 0.68 has been found post-treatment for psychological therapies in the treatment of depression

   d. CBT shows a slight superiority to short-term psychodynamic psychotherapy in the treatment of depression

   e. Short-term psychodynamic psychotherapy involves no more than 10 sessions (APT 2008)

19. The levels of attainment of psychodynamic formulation include all of the following except:

   a. Constructing an illness narrative

   b. Identifying transference

   c. Modelling a formulation

   d. Naming the elements

   e. Recognising the psychological dimension (APT 2006)

20. Which of the following statements about post-traumatic stress disorder is true?

   a. 25% of those suffering from it recover within 2 years

   b. Less than a third have a diagnosis after 6 years

   c. The lifetime prevalence is 2%

   d. It is associated with the male gender

   e. Over 50% of PTSD sufferers have another psychiatric disorder (APT 2007)

21. Which of the following statements about the neurobiology of PTSD is true?

a. The amygdala stores exact details of traumatic events

b. Patients with PTSD have high cortisol levels

c. The hippocampus mediates unconscious memories

d. PTSD represents a failure of the amygdala to regulate medial prefrontal activity

e. Small hippocampal volume is associated with PTSD (APT 2007)

22. All of the following statements about the treatment of PTSD are true except:

a. According to NICE, paroxetine is a second-line treatment for PTSD

b. Augmentation with olanzapine can be considered for treatment-resistant PTSD

c. Mirtazapine in the treatment of PTSD is associated with weight loss

d. NICE guidelines recommend that treatment should be considered for at least 1 year

e. Sertraline is indicated for the treatment of PTSD (APT 2007)

23. Which of the following statements about dependence on steroids is true?

a. Dependence is related to monoaminergic systems

b. Opioid use serves as a gateway for steroid use

c. Oral intake is the predominant route of administration

d. Sleepiness is a common withdrawal symptom

e. Around 10% of users trust information from drug dealers more than they trust information from doctors (APT 2006)

24. All of the following statements about the management of neuropsychiatric symptoms associated with hepatitis C are correct except:

    a. Anorexia responds well to paroxetine

    b. Gastrointestinal haemorrhage is known to be caused by antidepressants used for treating neuropsychiatric adverse effects from combination treatment

    c. Interferon-induced anxiety responds to SSRIs

    d. Naltrexone can be useful in the management of cognitive dysfunction

    e. Recombinant human erythropoietin has been useful in the treatment of apathy (APT under submission by the author)

25. All of the following statements about cognitive impairment and hepatitis C are true except:

    a. Abnormal P300 potentials have been seen in HCV infections

    b. The cognitive adverse effects of interferon include motor incoordination

    c. Cognitive impairment from interferon does not improve with the discontinuation of treatment

    d. Elevations in basal ganglia and white-matter choline/creatinine ratios have been found in HCV patients

    e. Impairment of verbal memory is a recognised adverse effect of interferon treatment (APT under submission by the author)

26. Which of the following statements about adverse neuropsychiatric effects of interferon treatment is true?

a. Apathy is the most common symptom

b. Anxiety is seen in 5% of patients who are on interferon

c. Its cognitive side-effects are suggestive of frontosubcortical impairment

d. Depression is seen in up to 10% of patients on interferon

e. The prevalence rate of adverse neuropsychiatric effects is up to 10% (APT under submission by the author)

27. Mrs Taylor presents with dizziness, double vision and difficulty in communication. The diagnosis is:

a. Acoustic neuroma

b. Benign paroxysmal positional vertigo

c. Labyrinthitis

d. Meniere's disease

e. Vertebrobasilar insufficiency (TN)

28. All of the following statements about treatment with ECT are true except:

a. Adverse psychological reactions are rare

b. It produces deficits in autobiographical and impersonal memory

c. The extent of retrograde amnesia is not significantly correlated with the degree of therapeutic improvement

d. Midazolam is contraindicated for patients who are agitated in the recovery phase from ECT

e. Its mortality risk is 1 per 10 000 patients (ECT)

29. Which of the following statements about the interaction between ECT and drug treatment is correct?

    a. Clozapine increases the seizure threshold

    b. Lithium increases the seizure threshold

    c. Olanzapine increases the seizure threshold

    d. SSRIs cause prolonged seizures

    e. Tricyclic antidepressants are anticonvulsant (ECT)

30. All of the following statements about ECT procedure are correct except:

    a. The extent of eventual improvement is associated with the improvement seen during the first few treatments

    b. In bilateral ECT, the initial treatment dose should be at least 100% more than that of the seizure threshold

    c. In unilateral ECT, the initial treatment dose should be at least 200% more than that of the seizure threshold

    d. The optimal technique for using unilateral ECT for mania has not been established

    e. The initial dose for male patients receiving unilateral ECT is 10% (ECT)

31. The tests of attention and concentration include all of the following except:

    a. The components of the Test of Everyday Attention

    b. The Corsi block-tapping span

    c. The Paused Auditory Serial Addition Test

    d. The reverse-digit span

    e. A timed test involving star cancellation (CA)

32. Which of the following is a test of personal memory?
    a. The cued word-association test
    b. The Doors and People Test
    c. Person-based tasks
    d. Tests of verbal knowledge
    e. Warrington's Recognition Memory Test (CA)

33. The hypothalamus forms the floor of the:
    a. Cerebellomedullary cistern
    b. Fourth ventricle
    c. Interventricular foramina of Munro
    d. Interpeduncular cistern
    e. Third ventricle (TN)

34. All of the following statements about the brain's blood supply are true except:
    a. All of the arteries that supply the brain are paired except for the basilar artery
    b. The carotid artery is flanked by the oculomotor and optic nerves
    c. The brain receives 750 mL of blood per minute
    d. The brain's large vessels are thin-walled
    e. A loss of blood supply for 10 to 15 seconds results in loss of consciousness (TN)

35. Mr Bainbridge presents with miosis, ptosis, vertigo, dysarthria and ipsilateral hemiataxia. This has been caused by stroke involving:

a. An aneurysm at the origin of the posterior communicating artery

b. The basilar artery

c. A Charcot–Bouchard aneurysm

d. The middle cerebral artery

e. The posterior inferior cerebellar artery (TN)

36. The sympathetic supply to the thyroid comes from the:

a. External carotid nerves

b. Inferior cervical ganglion

c. Internal carotid nerves

d. Middle cervical ganglion

e. Superior cervical ganglion (TN)

37. All of the following nerves include a parasympathetic component except:

a. III

b. V

c. VII

d. IX

e. X (TN)

38. All of the following statements about efferent fibres from the striatum are true except:

a. Fibres originate from the caudate nucleus

b. The striatonigral pathway uses substance P

c. The striatonigral fibres use acetylcholine

d. The striatopallidal fibres to the external segment use enkephalin

e. The striatopallidal fibres use glutamate as a neurotransmitter (TN)

39. Which of the following statements about cortico-thalamic-striatal circuits is true?

a. Their association loop involves the pars compacta of the substantia nigra

b. The head of the caudate is involved in the oculomotor loop

c. The lateral segment of the globus pallidus is involved in the limbic loop

d. The premotor cortex is part of the oculomotor loop

e. The ventrolateral nucleus of the thalamus connects to the supplementary motor cortex as part of the sensory–motor loop (TN)

40. All of the following matches with regard to the neurons in the basal ganglia are true except:

a. Intrastriatal interneurons – acetylcholinergic neurons that are inhibited by dopaminergic neurons

b. Neuropeptide-releasing neurons – release GABA and enkephalin from the same neuron

c. Pars compacta – neurons releasing dopamine have an excitatory effect on the GABA-ergic neurons that project to the lateral segment of the globus pallidus

d. Striatum – principally composed of GABA-releasing neurons

e. Subthalamic nucleus – gives rise to glutamate-releasing neurons (TN)

41. Mr Bainbridge presents with a lesion involving the ganglia branch of the left posterior cerebral artery. Which of the following statements is true?

a. Athetosis results from the degeneration of the medial segment of the globus pallidus

b. Dopaminergic agonists improve its symptoms

c. Left hypertonicity would be a feature

d. Primary degeneration of the GABA-ergic neurons ensues

e. Right hemiballismus would be a symptom (TN)

42. Mr Bainbridge presents with a wing-beating tremor that manifests following extension of an upper limb. In which of the following is this seen?

a. Friedreich's ataxia

b. Huntington's disease

c. Parkinson's disease

d. Sydenham's chorea

e. Wilson's disease (TN)

43. Which of the following statements about reflexes is true?

a. The afferent limb of the papillary light reflex is transmitted to the superior colliculus without synapsing at the lateral geniculate

b. The ciliospinal centre involved in the sympathetic pathway of the papillary dilation is situated at cord levels C1–C2

c. The efferent pathway of the blink reflex involves the nerve VII

d. In the convergence accommodation pathway, the inferior colliculus sends fibres to the Perlia's nucleus of the oculomotor complex

e. The pretectal area sends bilateral projections to the Edinger–Westphal nucleus (TN)

44. Which of the following is caused by a lesion of Myer's loop?

    a. Contralateral homonymous hemianopsia

    b. Contralateral upper homonymous quadrantopsia

    c. Contralateral lower homonymous quadrantopsia

    d. Contralateral homonymous hemianopsia with macular sparing

    e. Ipsilateral nasal hemianopsia (TN)

45. All of the following statements about auditory pathways are true except:

    a. First-order neurons are bipolar

    b. Fibres from the posteroventral cochlear nucleus terminate in the ventral nucleus of the lateral lemniscus

    c. Hair-receptor cells stimulate the peripheral process of first-order neurons

    d. Inferior olivary nuclei are involved in processing sound frequency

    e. The sound attenuation reflex involves the motor nucleus of the trigeminal nerve (TN)

46. All of the following cause conduction deafness except:

    a. Cerumen

    b. Jervell–Lange–Nielsen syndrome

    c. Otitis media

    d. Otosclerosis

    e. Perforation of the tympanic membrane (TN)

47. All of the following statements about nystagmus are true except:

   a. Extensive damage at the pontomedullary junction causes rotator nystagmus

   b. Horizontal nystagmus is normal

   c. The normal duration of post-rotatory nystagmus during a rotation test is half a minute

   d. Spontaneous nystagmus indicates a lesion affecting the vestibular nuclei

   e. Vertical nystagmus results from damage to the inferior vestibular nucleus (TN)

48. Mr Bainbridge presents with an inability to recognise complex sounds. Which of the following does the lesion involve?

   a. The bilateral primary auditory area

   b. The bilateral auditory association area

   c. The dominant auditory association area

   d. The dominant primary auditory area

   e. The non-dominant primary auditory area (TN)

49. A unilateral lesion to his non-dominant hemisphere will lead Mr Bainbridge to present specifically with which of the following?

   a. Amusia

   b. Auditory agnosia

   c. Partial deafness

   d. Receptive aphasia

   e. Total deafness (TN)

50. Mr Bainbridge has received a head injury leading to damage to his non-dominant cerebral hemisphere. All of the following domains will be impaired except:

    a. Mathematical skills

    b. Musical skills

    c. Poetry skills

    d. Recognition of faces

    e. Spatial perception (TN)

51. Which of the following processes is mediated by the dominant hemisphere?

    a. Music

    b. Poetry

    c. Problem solving

    d. Face recognition

    e. Spatial perception (TN)

52. All of the following statements about the middle cerebral artery are true except:

    a. An infarction of its more posterior branches is associated with visual agnosias

    b. It supplies both Broca's and Wernicke's areas

    c. It does not supply a narrow territory close to the sagittal fissure

    d. It supplies the medial surface of the brain

    e. It forms part of the circle of Willis (SBN)

53. All of the following types of receptors activate G-protein-coupled mechanisms except:

   a. A_2

   b. α_2

   c. D_1

   d. $GABA_B$

   e. $5\text{-}HT_4$ (SBN)

54. Which of the following neurotransmitter receptors is fast-ion-channel linked?

   a. Adenosine

   b. α_1

   c. Dopamine $_{2-4}$

   d. $GABA_B$

   e. $5\text{-}HT_3$ (SBN)

55. Which of the following statements about excitatory amino acids is true?

   a. At NMDA receptors, glutamate produces rapid trans-synaptic excitatory responses

   b. Glycine partial agonists increase NMDA function

   c. NMDA receptors are activated by phencyclidine

   d. Strychnine-insensitive glycine receptors modulate NMDA receptor function

   e. The synthesis of glutamate that functions as a transmitter is from glucose via Kreb's cycle (SBN)

56. Which of the following statements about GABA is true?

    a. The activators of GAD cause tonic seizures

    b. $GABA_A$ receptors presynaptically modulate GABA release

    c. Glutamic acid decarboxylase is a marker of GABA-ergic neurons

    d. Picrotoxin is an antagonist at the GABA receptor

    e. Schizophrenia may be related to decreased GABA activity (SBN)

57. Which of the following statements about acetylcholine is true?

    a. The action of acetylcholine is blocked by physostigmine

    b. The addictive aspects of nicotine are independent of dopaminergic systems

    c. Cholinergic processes are involved in NREM sleep

    d. Muscarinic receptors are not PI coupled

    e. The neuronal store of acetylcholine is depleted by hemicholinium (SBN)

58. Mr Bainbridge presents with a head injury, and you want to detect and measure the severity of visual neglect involved. Which of the following is the recommended test?

    a. The Behavioural Assessment of the Dysexecutive Syndrome

    b. The Behavioural Inattention Test

    c. The Delis–Kaplan Executive Function Syndrome

    d. The National Adult Reading Test

    e. Raven's Progressive Matrices (CA)

59. Mr Bainbridge presents with aphasia following a stroke. Which of the following can you use to measure his auditory comprehension?

a. The Rey Auditory Verbal Learning Test

b. The Rey–Osterrith Complex Figure Test

c. The Test for Reception of Grammar

d. The Token Test

e. The Trail Making Test (CA)

60. Mr Bainbridge presents with attentional deficits following a head injury. Which of the following will you use?

a. The Doors and People Test

b. The Judgement of Line Orientation Test

c. The Paced Auditory Serial Addition Test

d. The Recognition Memory Test

e. The Visual Object and Space Perception Battery (CA)

61. Mr Bainbridge has recovered from a head injury. Which of the following will you use to assess the extent of memory impairment recovered?

a. The National Adult Reading Test

b. The Pyramids and Palm Trees Test

c. Raven's Progressive Matrices

d. The Recognition Memory Test

e. The Rivermead Behavioural Memory Test (CA)

62. All of the following statements about the Cambridge Cognitive Examination are true except:

   a. It cannot distinguish different forms of dementias

   b. Its cut-off value for dementia is less than or equal to 80

   c. It forms part of CAMDEX

   d. The maximum score on CAMCOG is 100

   e. It is sensitive to mild dementia (CA)

63. Which of the following is associated with self-mutilation behaviour?

   a. Arnold–Chiari malformation

   b. De Lange malformation

   c. Generalised neurofibromatosis

   d. Tuberous sclerosis

   e. Von Hippel–Lindau disease (SBN)

64. All of the following statements about neural-tube defects are true except:

   a. Fetal ultrasound and amniotic fluid assay can identify 90% of defects *in vivo*

   b. Closure of the neural tube occurs within 18 to 26 days after the formation of the zygote

   c. In anencephaly, cerebral hemispheres fail to develop with exposure to diencephalon

   d. Minor neural-tube defects are present in less than 1% of the population without neurological deficits

   e. The recurrence rate for spina bifida in a second baby is 1 in 20 (SBN)

65. Which of the following statements about head injury is true?

    a. Being aged between 25 and 30 years is a risk factor for severe head injury

    b. The parietal lobe is the most vulnerable area for contusion damage

    c. Postconcussive symptoms usually resolve within 6 months

    d. Post-traumatic amnesia lasting 1 to 7 days is associated with mild sequelae

    e. The prevalence of severe disability following a head injury among the general population is 50 in 1 000 000 (SBN)

66. A neuropathological examination reveals anterior temporal cortical atrophy with balloon cells. In which of the following is this seen?

    a. Alzheimer's disease

    b. Creutzfeldt–Jacob disease

    c. Huntington's disease

    d. Parkinson's disease

    e. Pick's disease (SBN)

67. All of the following statements about Huntington's disease are true except:

    a. The cortical form of dementia is seen

    b. Choreiform movements become more pronounced as the disorder progresses

    c. Chromosome 4 is implicated in its aetiology

    d. The initial presentation is often psychiatric

    e. Its onset is usually in the third or fourth decade (SBN)

68. In which of the following is glucocerebrosidase deficiency seen?

   a. Gaucher's disease

   b. Gangliosidosis

   c. Leigh's disease

   d. Niemann–Pick disease

   e. Wilson's disease (SBN)

69. In which of the following is α-1-iduronidase deficiency seen?

   a. Hurler syndrome

   b. Hunter's syndrome

   c. Leigh's disease

   d. Niemann–Pick disease

   e. Tay–Sachs disease (SBN)

70. In which of the following leukodystrophies is X-linked recessive inheritance seen?

   a. Adrenoleukodystrophy

   b. Krabbe's leukodystrophy

   c. Metachromatic leukodystrophy

   d. Pelizaeus–Merzbacher disease

   e. Sudanophilic leukodystrophy (SBN)

71. Although leukodystrophies are characterised by the extensive degeneration of myelin, in which type of leukodytrophy can myelins be seen preserved around blood vessels?

   a. Adrenoleukodystrophy

   b. Krabbe's leukodystrophy

   c. Metachromatic leukodystrophy

   d. Pelizaeus–Merzbacher disease

   e. Sudanophilic leukodystrophy (SBN)

72. All of the following conditions are associated with demyelination except:

   a. Cyanocobalamin deficiency

   b. Leigh's disease

   c. Long-standing cerebral oedema

   d. Marchiafava–Bignami syndrome

   e. Progressive multifocal leucoencephalopathy (SBN)

73. The paraventricular nucleus is involved in controlling all of the following except:

   a. Corticotrophin-releasing hormone

   b. The dopamine-mediated inhibition of prolactin

   c. Somatostatin

   d. The stimulation of the secretion of growth hormone, mediated through GHRH

   e. Thyrotrophin-releasing hormone (SBN)

74. All of the following statements about growth hormone (GH) secretion are true except:

   a. Acetylcholine inhibits the release of somatostatin

   b. Growth hormone stimulates the peripheral production of IGF-1

   c. Nocturnal surges of GH occur during sleep stages 3 and 4

   d. Somatostatin has a direct inhibitory effect on GH secretion

   e. Stimulated GH secretion is lower in premenopausal women (SBN)

75. All of the following hormonal abnormalities are seen in anorexia nervosa except:

  a. Hypercortisolism with preserved diurnal rhythm

  b. Impaired gonadotrophin secretion

  c. Impaired osmotic regulation of arginine vasopressin

  d. Low total T_4

  e. Reduced growth-hormone response to levodopa (SBN)

76. Polyspikes and wave flattening are seen in:

  a. Absence seizures

  b. Atonic seizures

  c. Clonic seizures

  d. Tonic seizures

  e. Tonic–clonic seizures (SBN)

77. A regular and symmetrical 3 Hz pattern is seen in:

  a. Absence seizures

  b. Atonic seizures

  c. Clonic seizures

  d. Tonic seizures

  e. Tonic–clonic seizures (SBN)

78. The lifetime risk of unipolar depression among monozygotic co-twins of a bipolar proband is:

  a. 0.5–1.5%

  b. 2–5%

  c. 6–9%

  d. 10–13%

  e. 15–25% (PG)

79. All of the following statements about the genetic inheritance of bipolar affective disorder are true except:

a. An allele of a VNTR in intron 2 of the hSERT gene has been implicated in bipolar disorder

b. Chromosome 12q23-q24 has a LOD score of 2–0-4.9

c. Individuals with trisomy 21 are more susceptible to mania than the general population

d. A co-segregation of colour blindness and bipolar affective disorder exists

e. Tyrosine hydroxylase maps to 11p15 are implicated in bipolar disorder (PG)

80. All of the following statements about the genetics of bipolar affective disorder are true except:

a. Lithium responsiveness appears to be familial

b. A low-activity allele involving COMT polymorphism may be associated with increased susceptibility to rapid cycling

c. Gene coding for the 5-HT$_{2a}$ receptor has been implicated in rapid cycling disorder

d. The serotonin transporter gene (hSERT) has been implicated in seasonal affective disorder

e. Trinucleotide repeat expansion involving CTG18.1 has been implicated in bipolar disorder (PG)

81. The lifetime risk of schizophrenia-related psychosis among fraternal twins of patients with schizophrenia is:

a. 6%

b. 9%

c. 13%

d. 17%

e. 48% (PG)

82. The lifetime risk of developing schizophrenia-related psychosis among the grandchildren of patients with schizophrenia is:

a. 2%

b. 4%

c. 5%

d. 6%

e. 9% (PG)

83. Which of the following is an agonist at the 5-HT1A receptor?

a. Buspirone

b. Ergotamine

c. LSD

d. Methiothepin

e. Sumatriptan (N)

84. Which of the following statements about acetylcholine is true?

a. Acetylcholine produces long-term potentiation in the hippocampus by opening the K_M channels

b. All of the pathways of the autonomic system use acetylcholine as a neurotransmitter except for the preganglionic neurons

c. Cholinergic interneurons are absent in the nucleus accumbens

d. The laterodorsal tegmental nucleus is an important cholinergic pathway for regulating sleep and wakefulness

e. The motor neurons in the dorsal horn of the spinal cord are cholinergic (N)

85. All of the following statements about acetylcholine are true except:

a. The supply of acetyl CoA is the rate-limiting step in the synthesis of acetylcholine

b. The acetylcholine vesicle transporter is coded by the first exon of the ChAT gene

c. AChE enhances the response of cerebellar neurons to glutamate

d. The Na^+-dependent choline transporter is saturated at plasma choline concentrations

e. Nicotinic receptors mediate fast-ACh transmission, stimulating the dopamine-reward pathways (N)

86. Which of the following statements about purines is true?

a. A_1 receptors increase cAMP levels

b. Adenosine mediates the deleterious effects of oxidative stress on neurons

c. ATP acts as a transmitter in the CA3 region of the hippocampus

d. ATP is synaptically activated by an ecto-5'-nucleotidase

e. The $P_{2y}{}^a$ receptor is an ionotropic cation channel (N)

87. All of the following statements about peptide and tachykinin neurotransmission are true except:

a. The mRNA encoding a peptide neurotransmitter is transcripted on ribosomes

b. Peptides containing vesicles are moved by motor proteins along microtubules

c. The release of substance P in peripheral terminals results in neurogenic inflammation

d. Substance P is an excitatory tachykinin

e. Substance P is the preferred ligand for the NK1 receptor (N)

88. The enzyme used in the polymerase chain reaction is:

a. DNA trinucleotidase

b. Restriction endonuclease

c. Reverse transcriptase

d. RNA polymerase

e. Taq polymerase (PG)

89. A micro-array is called:

a. A DNA chip

b. A polymerase chain reaction

c. A primer extension

d. A restriction fragment length polymorphism

e. A short tandem repeat polymorphism (PG)

90. Mr Bainbridge cannot copy an image shown to him. This form of agnosia is:

a. Apperceptive agnosia

b. Associative agnosia

c. Autatopagnosia

d. Colour agnosia

e. Mirror agnosia (CA)

91. NF-1 is caused by a mutation of a gene on the long arm of chromosome:

a. 1

b. 9

c. 11

d. 15

e. 17 (KS)

92. The following are true regarding variant Creutzfeldt–Jakob disease except:

    a. Absence of periodic sharp waves on EEG

    b. Delayed neurological signs

    c. Marked accumulation of protease-resistant prion protein

    d. Mean age at death 60 years

    e. Pulvinar sign in more than 75% of cases (SBN)

93. Which of the following statements about cognitive-stimulation therapy in dementia is true?

    a. CST improves cognition but not depression

    b. It is composed only of reality orientation

    c. CST benefits quality of life but not cognition

    d. RCT evidence is available indicating that social groups improve cognition

    e. A high probability exists that CST is more cost-effective than treatment as usual (BJP 2006)

94. Which of the following statements about comorbid substance misuse and schizophrenia is true?

    a. Comorbid substance use and less severe negative symptoms have been reported

    b. IQ is not associated with an early age of onset of illness among substance misusers

    c. A negative correlation exists between cannabis use in adolescence and the development of schizophrenia in adulthood

    d. Stimulants and hallucinogens are the most commonly used substances among people who present with schizophrenia

    e. Substance misuse is a risk factor for relapse but not for onset (BJP 2006)

95. Which of the following statements about complementary medicines is true?

   a. Around 5–10% of all psychiatric patients rely on complementary medicines

   b. Around 10% of all cancer patients take psychoactive substances

   c. Evidence is available that melatonin can treat tardive dyskinesia

   d. Passionflower is potentially useful as a sedative

   e. Evidence is lacking that selenium complements antidepressant treatment (BJP 2006)

96. Increased bleeding time is associated with:

   a. Ginkgo

   b. Hydergine

   c. Panax ginseng

   d. Solanaceous plants

   e. Valerian (BJP 2006)

97. Which of the following drugs interacts with cholinesterase inhibitors?

   a. Ginkgo

   b. Hydergine

   c. Panax ginseng

   d. Solanaceous plants

   e. Valerian (BJP 2006)

98. Which of the following statements about the 5-HTTLPR genotype is true?

  a. The SERT-s allele is associated with a 25% reduction in volume of the anterior cingulate

  b. The SERT-l allele is associated with a 25% reduction in volume of the amygdala

  c. Suicide is dependent upon major depression for contributing to the enlargement of the thalamus

  d. The 5-HTTLPR genotype is associated with a 20% reduction in the number of neurons in the pulvinar nucleus

  e. The history of antidepressant treatment is associated with an increase in thalamic volume (BJP 2008)

99. Which of the following statements about attribution style and depression is true?

  a. Attributional style is not a mediator of the genetic influences on depression

  b. Attributional style is unrelated to current mood

  c. People who are experiencing their first episode of depression are more likely to attribute it to an internal cause than people who are experiencing recurrent depression

  d. People who are likely to view the causes of events as global are less likely to develop depression in future

  e. People who are likely to view the causes of negative events as internal are less likely to develop depression in future (BJP 2008)

100. Which of the following statements about neural circuits in OCD is true?

   a. Adults with OCD perform well on motor and interference inhibition but not on task switching

   b. A dysfunction of the frontocerebellar attention networks is evident during the cognitive forms of inhibition

   c. fMRIs show that inhibition failure in adolescents with OCD is associated with mesial frontal over-activation

   d. Frontostriatal over-activation is seen during inhibitory tasks

   e. An improvement in impaired inhibitory performance is a marker of symptom improvement (BJP 2008)

101. All of the following statements about CBT are true except:

   a. A 12-week comprehensive treatment programme consisting of CBT, body awareness therapy and graded exercise is more effective than antidepressant therapy in chronic fatigue syndrome

   b. According to the Nottingham Study of Neurotic Disorder, cognitive therapy and self-help were more effective for depressed people with comorbid personality disorder than for people without personality disorder

   c. CBT with a problem-solving component has a positive effect on self-harm

   d. People with a personality disorder who respond to cognitive therapy show sustained responses

   e. Schema-focused therapy has been found to reduce self-harm in patients with borderline personality disorder (BJP 2008)

102. All of the following statements about schizophrenia are true except:

    a. Any craniofacial/midline anomaly is associated with an increased risk of schizophrenia-spectrum disorder

    b. Febrile seizures are not associated with adult schizophrenia

    c. Impaired extrastriate visual processing of fear is associated with negative symptoms

    d. Increased semantic priming is associated with thought disorders

    e. The recognition of negative facial affect is impaired in people with schizophrenia (BJP 2008)

103. Which of the following statements about schizophrenia is true?

    a. Atypical antipsychotics are more effective than typical antipsychotics in the treatment of delusional parasitosis

    b. Cognitive remediation therapy is not associated with durable improvements in working memory

    c. Fewer than 1% of the people who harm themselves die in the subsequent year

    d. Patients with positive symptoms show a higher degree of impairment of their mentalisation than do disorganised patients

    e. Population density interacts with poor pre-morbid cognitive functioning (BJP 2007)

104. All of the following influence caregiver stress in schizophrenia except:

    a. The caregiver being the patient's parent

    b. The highest burden being in relation to the supervision of the patient

    c. The patient being male

    d. The patient's marital status

    e. The patient's symptoms (BJP 2007)

105. Which of the following statements about schizophrenia is true?

a. Awareness of the illness is associated more with impaired working memory

b. Cortical microstructure disruption is seen in the temporo-occipital lobes

c. Motor-cortex reactions are weaker in both patients and their twin siblings

d. Patients who use cannabis show normal anterior cingulate, in contrast to those who do not use it

e. Age has a positive effect on the integrity of the left superior longitudinal fasciculus (BJP 2007)

106. All of the following statements about depression are true except:

a. Ceasing to cohabit with a partner precipitates depression

b. ECT is the most effective treatment for depression

c. ECT patients are more medically ill

d. Personality disorders affect outcomes in depressed people who are being treated with interpersonal therapy

e. rTMS augments antidepressant treatment (BJP 2007)

107. Which of the following statements about PTSD is true?

a. Basal cortisol levels are low in morning samples

b. Cortisol activates neuronal defensive reactions

c. Serotonin from the amygdala inhibits the hypothalamus from secreting corticotrophin-releasing hormone

d. Sexual abuse is associated with higher basal cortisol levels

e. Trauma-focused CBT is as effective as EMDR (BJP 2007)

108. Which of the following statements about neuroleptic malignant syndrome (NMS) is true?

a. Bromocriptine, but not amantadine, reduces its mortality rate

b. Dantrolene takes 24 hours to produce a clinical effect

c. Its mortality rate is less than 10% with NMS from depot antipsychotic medications

d. Its prevalence is 0.02–2.4%

e. Untreated symptoms resolve within 7 days (KS)

109. Mr Bainbridge presents with hyperthermia, muscle rigidity, palpitation, hypotension, rhabdomyolysis and disseminated intra-vascular coagulation. This can be caused by:

a. Amphetamine

b. Atropine

c. Lead poisoning

d. Reserpine

e. Succinylcholine (KS)

110. In which of the following are β-adrenergic antagonists definitely effective?

a. Adjunctive therapy for alcohol withdrawal

b. Adjunctive therapy for aggressive behaviour

c. Antidepressant augmentation

d. Antipsychotic augmentation

e. Lithium-induced tremor (KS)

111. The adverse effects of β-adrenergic receptor antagonists include all of the following except:

    a. Diarrhoea

    b. Hypotension

    c. Hyperglycaemia

    d. Impotence

    e. Peyronie's disease (KS)

112. All of the following statements about amantadine are true except:

    a. Amantadine coadministered with MAOIs can cause a significant increase in blood pressure ·

    b. Amantadine is contraindicated in people who are sensitive to anticholinergic effects

    c. Amantadine has benefits in the treatment of ejaculatory inhibition

    d. Amantadine is excreted unmetabolised in urine

    e. Livedo reticularis has been seen in 5% of people taking amantadine (KS)

113. All of the following statements about psychotic symptoms among the general population are true except:

    a. An excess of apparent hallucinations has been reported among men compared with women

    b. Established psychotic symptoms may be present in milder forms in the general population

    c. A 1-year incidence of around 5% has been reported for hallucinations among the general population

    d. Similarities exist between the risk factors for psychotic symptoms and schizophrenia among the general population

    e. An association exists between baseline neurosis and incident psychotic symptoms among the general population (BJP 2006)

114. All of the following are risk factors for self-reported psychotic symptoms among the general population except:

    a. Harmful pattern of drinking

    b. Living in an urban area

    c. More adverse life events

    d. Having a small primary support group

    e. Smoking tobacco (BJP 2006)

115. All of the following statements about the risk factors for psychiatric illnesses among women from low-income countries are true except:

    a. Being married

    b. Living in a relatively large household

    c. Poverty

    d. Reporting chronic physical illnesses

    e. Use of tobacco (BJP 2006)

116. The risk factors for severe postpartum psychosis include all of the following except:

    a. Caesarean section

    b. Delivery complications

    c. Delivering a female baby

    d. Multiparity

    e. Having a relatively shorter gestation period (BJP 2006)

117. All of the following statements about the neuropathology of hallucinations are true except:

    a. Hallucinations increase N100 in amplitude

    b. The primary auditory cortex is involved

    c. Reduced left temporal responsivity is present

    d. The right cortical area is the most important one for direction discrimination

    e. When Broca's area alone dominates, inner speech is perceived (BJP 2007)

118. Dysthymic disorder has a prevalence of:

    a. 0.5–1%

    b. 1–3%

    c. 3–6%

    d. 7–8%

    e. 9–14% (KS)

119. The lifetime prevalence of hypomania is:

    a. 0–1.2%

    b. 1.2–2.4%

    c. 2.6–7.8%

    d. 8–12.5%

    e. 12.8–14.8% (KS)

120. All of the following statements about gender differences between affective disorders are true except:

    a. Bipolar type 1 disorder has a higher prevalence among men

    b. Manic episodes are more common in men

    c. Major depressive disorders are twice as prevalent in women as in men

    d. There is a higher rate of rapid cyclers among women

    e. Women present with a more mixed picture than men when presenting with a manic episode (KS)

121. All of the following are indicators of a good prognosis in depression except:

    a. The absence of a comorbid personality disorder

    b. Early age of onset

    c. Having had no more than one previous hospitalisation

    d. A relatively short hospital stay

    e. Having had strong friendships during adolescence (KS)

122. Which of the following statements about the course of bipolar disorder is true?

    a. Bipolar type 1 disorder most often starts with mania

    b. The incidence of bipolar disorder in children and adolescents is about 1%

    c. Fewer than 5% of people with bipolar disorder can be classified as rapid cyclers

    d. Around 15% of patients with bipolar type 1 disorder do not have a recurrence of symptoms

    e. Around 30% of patients with bipolar disorder achieve significant control over their symptoms with lithium (KS)

123. Positive relationship transference without interpretation is a technique used in which of the following?

    a. Brief psychodynamic approach

    b. Cognitive behavioural therapy

    c. Dialectical behaviour therapy

    d. Interpersonal therapy

    e. Psychodynamic therapy (KS)

124. Therapists associated with interpersonal therapy include all of the following except:

    a. Jacobson

    b. Klerman

    c. Meyer

    d. Sullivan

    e. Weissman (KS)

125. All of the following are the patient variables most suited for interpersonal therapy except:

    a. A focused dispute with a partner or significant other

    b. A modest to moderate need for direction and guidance

    c. Pragmatic thinking

    d. Responsiveness to environmental manipulation

    e. Social or communication problems (KS)

126. Which of the following is the confirmation of reality by comparing one's own conceptualisations with those of other members in the group?
    a. Acceptance
    b. Cohesion
    c. Consensual validation
    d. Corrective family experience
    e. Reality testing (KS)

127. Self-disclosure is also known as:
    a. Catharsis
    b. Contagion
    c. Empathy
    d. Transference
    e. Ventilation (KS)

128. Which of the following is the process during which the group leader formulates the meaning or significance of a patient's resistance?
    a. Acceptance
    b. Consensual validation
    c. Identification
    d. Interpretation
    e. Reality testing (KS)

129. The roles in a psychodrama include all of the following except:
    a. Auxiliary ego
    b. Director
    c. Group
    d. Narrator
    e. Protagonist (KS)

130. Which of the following types of family therapy emphasises individual maturation in the context of the family system and is free from unconscious patterns of anxiety and projection rooted in the past?

    a. Bowen model

    b. General systems model

    c. Psychodynamic–experiential model

    d. Social network model

    e. Structural model (KS)

3

Paper 3

1. Which of the following statements about the neuropathology of premenstrual syndrome is true?

   a. Basal plasma and urinary cortisol levels do not distinguish women with premenstrual syndrome from controls

   b. Its estimated heritability is approximately 20%

   c. The exacerbation of serotonergic activity by tryptophan manifests as premenstrual syndrome

   d. Patients' levels of allopregnanolone increase after treatment with antidepressants, suggesting a causal pathway involving the GABA system

   e. Lower β-endorphin levels are found in the luteal phase only (APT 2007)

2. Which of the following statements about the epidemiology of the antidepressant discontinuation syndrome is true?

   a. Of the SSRIs, paroxetine is least associated with discontinuation symptoms

   b. A study with venlafaxine showed that approximately 25% of the sample developed discontinuation symptoms

   c. Its symptoms are less common when higher doses are discontinued

   d. Its symptoms are not associated with the duration of the treatment

   e. Clinical studies show no difference between gradual and abrupt discontinuation (APT 2007)

3. The basic principles of motivational interviewing include all of the following except:

   a. Express empathy

   b. Develop discrepancy

   c. Reward reflections

   d. Roll with resistance

   e. Support self-efficacy (APT 2008)

4. The components of a relapse prevention programme include all of the following except:

   a. The creation of a self-help sheet

   b. Identifying alternative pleasurable activities

   c. The management of anger using problem-solving techniques

   d. Rewarding reflections

   e. Role play (APT 2008)

5. All of the following statements about the neuropathology of catatonia are true except:

   a. The presence of abnormal metabolism in the thalamus and frontal lobes

   b. The bottom-up modulation of the basal ganglia due to a deficiency of GABA

   c. Clozapine-withdrawal catatonia is due to cholinergic and serotonergic rebound hyperactivity

   d. A dysfunction in glutamate

   e. A sudden block of dopamine receptors (APT 2007)

6. Which of the following statements about the diagnosis and classification of catatonia is true?

   a. The Bush–Francis Catatonia Rating Scale aids in distinguishing between catatonia and extrapyramidal symptoms

   b. Ictal catatonia is due to the involvement of the temporal lobe

   c. Catatonia is more commonly a consequence of a mood disorder than of schizophrenia

   d. Catatonia due to physical causes is diagnosed as other catatonic disorder according to ICD-10

   e. Systematic catatonia is linked to chromosome site 15q15 (APT 2007)

7. All of the following statements about the treatment of catatonia are true except:

   a. Antipsychotics precipitate neuroleptic malignant syndrome in patients with catatonia

   b. Death due to pulmonary embolism is more common in the second week

   c. Organic catatonia responds to benzodiazepines

   d. Patients who do not respond to benzodiazepines require ECT

   e. Recurrence rates are higher for catatonia from schizophrenia than that from affective disorders (APT 2007)

8. Which of the following statements about the neurodevelopmental aspects of schizophrenia is true?

   a. A combination of risperidone and CBT has been found to be effective in people at risk of the development of psychosis

   b. Delayed developmental milestones are a specific neurodevelopmental precursor of schizophrenia

   c. Environmental interventions in childhood do not have a positive impact on reducing schizotypy in later life

   d. Impaired cognitive functioning is not related to early onset

   e. Obstetric complication is not associated with poorer outcomes (APT 2007)

9. Which of the following statements about first-episode psychosis is true?

   a. Attenuated symptoms is a category under trait factors according to the Melbourne criteria

   b. Cannabis use does not promote psychotic experiences in people without a pre-existing vulnerability

   c. A change in mental state lasting at least 1 month is a state character

   d. Only 10% of the general population identified as cases using the Bonn Scale for the Assessment of Basic Symptoms go on to develop a disorder

   e. The rate of transition to psychosis using the Melbourne criteria has been reported to be between 28% and 40% (APT 2006)

10. Which of the following statements about the management of people at risk of psychosis is true?

    a. Delays in access to early-intervention services are due to the ego-dystonic nature of the symptoms

    b. High scores on the GAF are a predictor of progress towards psychosis

    c. A 1-year treatment with olanzapine offers a significant advantage

    d. Risperidone at a low dose combined with CBT and needs-based intervention prevents the onset of psychosis

    e. A significant lowering of the transition rate is associated with CBT (APT 2006)

11. All of the following are tasks that could be used to measure every-day memory functioning in patients receiving ECT except:

    a. The Autobiographical Memory Index

    b. The Everyday Memory Interview

    c. The nine-point mood rating scale

    d. The landmark location task

    e. The virtual map task (APT 2007)

12. All of the following are recommended elements of a cognitive rehabilitative programme for ECT except:

    a. A comprehensive neuropsychological assessment

    b. Feedback to the patient and family

    c. Psychoeducation for the patient and caregiver

    d. Strategy learning focusing on decompensation

    e. The transfer of acquired skills to all domains of the patient's life (APT 2007)

13. MRI evidence suggests that patients with multiple sclerosis who exhibit mania with psychotic symptoms have plaques in:

    a. The dorso-lateral frontal cortex

    b. The non-dominant parietal lobe

    c. The orbitofrontal cortex

    d. The pre-frontal cortex

    e. The temporal horn (APT 2006)

14. All of the following drugs have been used for the treatment of pathological laughing and crying in multiple sclerosis except:

    a. Amantadine

    b. Amitryptyline

    c. Carbamazepine

    d. Fluoxetine

    e. Levodopa (APT 2006)

15. The drug for which there is evidence with regard to treating cognitive impairment in multiple sclerosis is:

    a. Donepezil

    b. Galantamine

    c. Memantine

    d. Rivastigmine

    e. None of the above (APT 2006)

16. All of the following statements about the epidemiology of Munchausen's syndrome are true except:

   a. Nearly a quarter of the people with Munchausen's syndrome have been working in occupations associated with the medical profession

   b. Simple fictitious disorders involve health workers in their thirties

   c. The typical onset is below the age of 30 years

   d. Being an unmarried male is an indicator of severe Munchausen's syndrome

   e. Women are more frequently affected than men (APT 2008)

17. Which of the following statements about the diagnosis of Munchausen's disease is true?

   a. The absence of visits by family members has been proposed to be of diagnostic significance

   b. Asher described three types of psychological manifestations

   c. Cutaneous type was one of the subtypes proposed by Asher

   d. DSM-IV categorises Munchausen's disease into physical, psychological and mixed subtypes

   e. The dyad of Munchausen's disease involves pseudologia fantastica but not peregrination (APT 2008)

18. All of the following statements about PTSD are correct except:

   a. A genetic factor has been shown to account for 34% of cases of PTSD

   b. High levels of neuropeptide Y have been found in combat veterans with PTSD

   c. Increased levels of corticotrophin-releasing hormone are found in the CSF of patients with PTSD

   d. Numbing is strongly associated with chronicity

   e. The prevalence of PTSD among people directly affected by terrorism is between 12% and 16% (APT 2007)

19. Which of the following statements about PTSD is correct?

a. It involves decreased platelet 5-hydroxy tryptamine levels

b. It involves decreased plasma dopamine levels

c. It involves diminished glucocorticoid-receptor sensitivity

d. The DRD2 gene is associated with comorbid psychosis with PTSD

e. The hyper-suppression of cortisol with dexamethasone suppression test is indicated (APT 2007)

20. Which of the following statements about schizophrenia and violence is correct?

a. Approximately 5% of those found guilty of non-fatal violence have schizophrenia

b. The annual risk that a patient with schizophrenia will commit homicide is 1 in 10 000

c. Fewer than 5% of those awaiting trial for murder have a schizophrenic disorder

d. Minor forms of assault are more common in schizophrenia, at 20% per year

e. Schizophrenia is five times more common among prisoners than in the general population (APT 2006)

21. Which of the following statements about the diagnosis of bipolar affective disorder is true?

    a. Approximately 10% of patients with bipolar affective disorder have been diagnosed with schizophrenia

    b. About 25% of patients with depression have irritable mood

    c. Bipolar type 2 disorder is the only major DSM-IV syndrome not associated with significant social or occupational dysfunction

    d. Bipolar type 2 disorder is more common than bipolar type 1 disorder

    e. Only about 50% of patients with a diagnosis of bipolar affective disorder have ever been treated on monotherapy with a mood stabiliser (www.psychiatrycpd.co.uk)

22. Polypharmacy in schizophrenia is associated with all of the following except:

    a. Approximately 15% of patients being discharged on antipsychotic polypharmacy

    b. An increase in at least one adverse event

    c. The increasing fragmentation of services

    d. Long-term antipsychotic polypharmacy during the year after discharge being less than 5%

    e. A prevalence as high as 50% among inpatients (www.psychiatrycpd.co.uk)

23. All of the following statements about the management of falls are true except:

    a. According to the Cochrane Review, multifactor risk assessment is one of the effective factors for the management of falls

    b. Cardiogenic syncope is more likely to be fatal than neurogenic syncope

    c. Fludrocortisone is used as an option in the management of postural hypotension when non-pharmacological measures fail

    d. One of the aims of the NSF is to provide advice on prevention through a specialised falls service

    e. There is robust evidence supporting the use of hip protectors to prevent fractures in community populations (www.psychiatrycpd.co.uk)

24. All the following increase urinary frequency without retention except:

    a. Alcohol

    b. Benzodiazepines

    c. Caffeine

    d. Calcium-channel blockers

    e. Diuretics (www.psychiatrycpd.co.uk)

25. All of the following matches with regard to ECT and age are correct except:

    a. Adult – posterior beta

    b. Adult – anterior alpha

    c. Infant – low amplitude

    d. Old age – decrease in delta

    e. 2–6 years – mature rhythms (SBN)

26. As which of the following do focal cerebral lesions show on the EEG?

   a. Dominant theta

   b. Normal record with fast activity

   c. Slow rhythms

   d. Spike and wave pattern

   e. Unreactive delta (SBN)

27. In which of the following is frontal intermittent rhythmic delta activity seen?

   a. Alzheimer's disease

   b. Metabolic encephalopathy

   c. Myoclonic epilepsy

   d. Presenile dementias

   e. Renal encephalopathy (SBN)

28. Which of the following does the neural basis of phonology involve?

   a. The anterior temporal lobe

   b. Broca's area

   c. The inferior temporal lobe

   d. The left anterior hemisphere

   e. The left superior temporal lobe (CA)

29. In which of the following are the basal ganglia involved?

   a. Phonology

   b. Prosody

   c. Semantics

   d. Syntax

   e. None of the above (CA)

30. Lesions posterior to the sylvian fissure cause difficulties in:

    a. Comprehension

    b. Fluency

    c. Naming

    d. Repetition

    e. All of the above (CA)

31. In which of the following aphasic syndromes is repetition pre-served?

    a. Broca's

    b. Conduction

    c. Global

    d. Transcortical motor

    e. Wernicke's (CA)

32. Which of the following is a word–picture matching test of single-word comprehension?

    a. The Beach Scene Test

    b. The Boston Diagnostic Aphasia Examination

    c. The Boston Naming and Graded Naming Test

    d. The Doors and People Test

    e. The Peabody Picture Vocabulary Test (CA)

33. Mr Bainbridge presents with miosis, ptosis, anhydrosis and eno-phthalmos. Which of the following is the possible cause?

    a. Horner's syndrome

    b. Lambert–Eaton syndrome

    c. Shy–Drager syndrome

    d. Wallenberg syndrome

    e. All of the above (TN)

34. In Lambert–Eaton syndrome, against which of the following are antibodies produced?

a. The acetylcholinesterase enzyme

b. The acetylcholine transporter

c. The muscarinic receptors

d. The nicotinic receptors

e. The voltage-gated calcium channels (TN)

35. All of the following types of receptors show slow adaptation except:

a. The Golgi tendon organs

b. Merkel's tactile discs

c. Nociceptors

d. Peritrichial nerve endings

e. Ruffini's organs (TN)

36. Which of the following receptors sends nerve fibres through the anterolateral system?

a. Free nerve endings

b. Merkel's tactile discs

c. Meissner's corpuscles

d. Pacinian corpuscles

e. Peritrichial nerve endings (TN)

37. With which of the following are Aα myelinated fibres associated?

a. The Golgi tendon organs

b. Merkel's tactile discs

c. Nociceptors

d. Peritrichial nerve endings

e. Ruffini's organs (TN)

38. All of the following are cerebellar nuclei except:

a. Dentate

b. Emboliform

c. Fastigius

d. Globose

e. Red (TN)

39. Taurine is used as a neurotransmitter in the cerebellum by which of the following cell types?

a. Basket

b. Granule

c. Inner stellate

d. Outer stellate

e. Purkinje (TN)

40. Which of the following cell types in the cerebellum is excitatory?

a. Basket

b. Golgi

c. Granule

d. Outer stellate

e. Purkinje (TN)

41. All of the following statements about the lobes of the cerebellum are true except:

a. The anterior lobe is the spinocerebellum

b. The flocculonodular lobe consists of the pontocerebellum

c. The posterior lobe is also known as the neocerebellum

d. The posterior lobe is involved with non-stereotype skilled movement

e. The vermis is part of the anterior lobe (TN)

42. The efferent fibres that pass through the superior cerebellar peduncle include all of the following except:

   a. The cerebelloreticular fibres

   b. The dentatorubrothalamic pathway

   c. The fastigiothalamic tract

   d. The fastigiovestibular tract

   e. The interpositorubrothalamic pathway (TN)

43. Which of the following statements about the olfactory pathway
is true?

   a. The medial olfactory stria is the main central pathway of the
olfactory system

   b. The olfactory bulbs are outgrowths of the metencephalon

   c. The olfactory receptor cells give rise to myelinated axons

   d. The olfactory tract carries both afferent and efferent fibres

   e. The primary olfactory cortex projects to the
ventroposteromedial nucleus of the thalamus (TN)

44. All of the following statements about the limbic system are true
except:

   a. The dentate gyrus is part of the archicortex

   b. The hippocampus forms a prominence on the lateral wall of
the inferior horn of the lateral ventricle

   c. The output target of the hippocampus includes the
mammillary body

   d. The subcallosal gyri form a part of it

   e. The polymorphic layer of the hippocampus consists of
interneurons (TN)

45. Which of the following statements about the hippocampus is true?

    a. CA2 zone cells are the primary cells contributing to the memory process through long-term potentiation

    b. The cingulate gyrus connects the hippocampus to the hypothalamus

    c. The entorhinal cortex provides major input to the hippocampal formation

    d. The hippocampal archicortex consists of four layers

    e. A lesion of the hippocampal formation causes an inability to retrieve information from long-term memory (TN)

46. The production of oxytocin and ADH is under the control of:

    a. The preoptic nucleus

    b. The medial preoptic nucleus

    c. The lateral preoptic nucleus

    d. The suprachiasmatic nucleus

    e. The supraoptic nucleus (TN)

47. Which of the following is the satiety centre?

    a. The arcuate nucleus

    b. The dorsomedial nucleus

    c. The periventricular nucleus

    d. The paraventricular nucleus

    e. The ventromedial nucleus (TN)

48. Which of the following statements about the ventricular system is true?

   a. The choroid plexus secretes 500 mL of CSF every day

   b. CSF is transported back into the ventricular system through the foramen of Luschka

   c. The aqueduct of Sylvius is situated above the tectum in the midbrain

   d. The body of the lateral ventricle is situated below the corpus callosum

   e. The fourth ventricle lies above the cerebellum (SBN)

49. Which of the following statements about the ascending sensory tracts is true?

   a. The affective component of pain appreciation is dependent on the somatosensory cortex

   b. The axons from the lumbar and sacral columns form the cuneate column

   c. The axons that branch to the dorsal horn mediate the polysynaptic reflexes

   d. The second-order neurons of the spinothalamic tract cross two segments above their spinal cord levels

   e. The second-order fibres that carry somaesthetic sensation from the head terminate in the inferior end of the postcentral gyrus (SBN)

50. Which of the following statements about the visual pathway is true?

    a. The fibres from the lower field pass to the superior bank of the calcarine fissure

    b. A homonymous defect in an upper quadrant of the visual field suggests a disorder of the ipsilateral temporal lobe

    c. The input to the superior colliculi serves as the efferent to visual avoidance reflexes

    d. The receptors synapse with the ganglion cells

    e. The rods outnumber the cones in all areas of the retina (SBN)

51. Which of the following statements about the hearing pathway is true?

    a. High-frequency sound is localised by the superior olivary nucleus

    b. The superior cochlear nuclei are situated around the inferior cerebellar peduncle

    c. The auditory pathway is entirely crossed

    d. The third-order neuron crosses in the midline in the trapezoid body

    e. Unilateral lesions of Heschl's gyrus are accompanied by unilateral deafness (SBN)

52. All of the following are characteristics of an upper motor neuron lesion except:

    a. The absence of superficial reflexes

    b. A Babinski sign

    c. Hypertonia

    d. Spastic paralysis

    e. Wasting (SBN)

53. Which of the following statements about dopamine is true?

    a. DOPA decarboxylase is the rate-controlling enzyme

    b. The extra-neuronal metabolism of dopamine is by COMT

    c. Increasing tyrosine increases the level of catecholamaines

    d. The nigrostriatal system has a higher turnover of dopamine than the mesolimbic system

    e. Plasma HVA shows a very long lag in its response to neuroleptics (SBN)

54. Which of the following statements about dopamine receptors is true?

    a. Apomorphine is their D_2-receptor antagonist

    b. Domperidone is their D_2-receptor antagonist

    c. Clozapine has a higher D_5-to-D_4 receptor binding

    d. Pergolide is their D_1-receptor agonist

    e. Sulpiride is their D_4-receptor antagonist (N)

55. Which of the following statements about noradrenaline is true?

    a. In the adrenal medulla, noradrenaline is converted to adrenaline by demethylation

    b. MHPG does not cross the blood–brain barrier

    c. The non-neuronal metabolism of noradrenaline occurs through MAO-A

    d. Noradrenaline is derived from dopamine by noradrenaline-β-hydroxylase

    e. Noradrenergic projection to the forebrain occurs in two bundles (SBN)

56. Which of the following statements about adrenergic receptors is true?

   a. Adrenaline is a stronger agonist as a β-receptor than is isoprenaline

   b. The $β_1$-receptors are rich in the cerebellum

   c. Prazosin is their $α_2$-antagonist

   d. Presynaptic $α_2$-receptors control the release of noradrenaline

   e. Yohimbine is their $α_2$-agonist (SBN)

57. Which of the following statements about serotonin is true?

   a. Platelets store 5% of the serotonin in the blood

   b. 5-HIAA has a lumbo-cervical concentration gradient

   c. Alanine competes for the same transmitter as tryptophan

   d. High levels of 5-HIAA are associated with arson

   e. Tryptophan hydroxylase is the rate limiter of synthesis (SBN)

58. Which of the following is the test of abstract behaviour?

   a. The Doors and People Test

   b. The National Adult Reading Test

   c. The Rivermead Behavioural Memory Test

   d. The Stroop Test

   e. The Wisconsin Card Sorting Test (CA)

59. Which of the following is a test of the right parietal lobe?

   a. The Boston Naming Test

   b. The Doors and People Test

   c. The Graded Naming Test

   d. The Hayling and Brixton test

   e. The Judgement of Line Orientation Test (CA)

60. Which of the following is a verbal subscale of WAIS-R?

    a. Block design

    b. Digit–symbol substitution

    c. Picture arrangement

    d. Picture completion

    e. Similarities (CA)

61. Which of the following is a performance subscale on WAIS?

    a. Arithmetic

    b. Digit span

    c. Digit–symbol substitution

    d. Information

    e. Vocabulary (CA)

62. Which of the following is not a WMS subscale?

    a. Digit span

    b. Information and orientation

    c. Logical memory

    d. Mental control

    e. Picture completion (CA)

63. All of the following are tests of the frontal lobe except:

    a. The Benton Verbal Fluency Test

    b. The Benton Visual Retention Test

    c. The Halstead Category Test

    d. The Trail Making Test

    e. The Wisconsin Card Sorting Test (SBN)

64. Which of the following is a specific test for spatial dyslexia and dyscalculia?

    a. The arithmetic scale of the Luria–Nebraska Battery

    b. The Rey Complex Figure

    c. The Left–Right Disorientation Test

    d. The Speech Sound Perception Test

    e. The Trail Making Test (SBN)

65. All of the following statements about head injuries are true except:

    a. The Galveston Orientation and Memory Test is a specific test of post-traumatic amnesia

    b. Neuropsychological assessment has a sensitivity of 90–95%

    c. The prognostic value of post-traumatic amnesia is most closely seen in closed and blunt head injuries

    d. Retrograde amnesia is a reliable index of the severity of brain damage but not of its prognosis

    e. Retrograde amnesia results from lacerations to the frontal and temporal regions (SBN)

66. All of the following are tests of language function except:

    a. The Benton Verbal Fluency Test

    b. The Boston Diagnostic Aphasia Examination

    c. Repeating 'no ifs, ands or buts' in Addenbrooke's Cognitive Examination

    d. The Rey Auditory Verbal Learning Test

    e. The Revised Token Test (SBN)

67. Which of the following is a test of laterality?

    a. The Dichotic Listening Test

    b. Finger Oscillation

    c. Finger-Tip Number Writing

    d. Right–Left Orientation

    e. The Trail Making Test (SBN)

68. In which of the following is vascular malformation of the retina seen?

    a. Bilateral acoustic neurofibromatosis

    b. Sturge–Weber syndrome

    c. Tuberous sclerosis

    d. von Hippel–Lindau disease

    e. von Recklinghausen's neurofibromatosis (SBN)

69. In which of the following is IgA deficiency seen?

    a. Ataxia telangiectasia

    b. Bilateral acoustic neurofibromatosis

    c. Sturge–Weber syndrome

    d. Tuberous sclerosis

    e. von Hippel–Lindau disease (SBN)

70. In which of the following is gene deletion on chromosome 22 seen?

    a. Ataxia telangiectasia

    b. Bilateral acoustic neurofibromatosis

    c. Sturge–Weber syndrome

    d. Tuberous sclerosis

    e. von Hippel–Lindau disease (SBN)

71. The autosomal dominant form of phakomatoses with an abnormality of chromosome 17 is called:
    a. Bilateral acoustic neurofibromatosis
    b. Sturge–Weber syndrome
    c. Tuberous sclerosis
    d. von Hippel–Lindau disease
    e. von Recklinghausen's neurofibromatosis (SBN)

72. Subungual angifibromas are seen in:
    a. Bilateral acoustic neurofibromatosis
    b. Sturge–Weber syndrome
    c. Tuberous sclerosis
    d. von Hippel–Lindau disease
    e. von Recklinghausen's neurofibromatosis (SBN)

73. High-amplitude clusters of mixed delta waves and multifocal spikes occurring particularly during sleep are characteristic of:
    a. Grand mal
    b. Hypsarrhythmia
    c. Lennox–Gastaut syndrome
    d. Myoclonus
    e. Petit mal (SBN)

74. Slow 2 Hz complexes with gradual cessation and the discharge enhancing in non-REM sleep are characteristic of:
    a. Grand mal
    b. Hypsarrhythmia
    c. Lennox–Gastaut syndrome
    d. Myoclonus
    e. Petit mal (SBN)

75. All of the following statements about cognitive-event-related potentials are true except:

  a. Attenuated cognitive negative variants have been reported in psychopathy

  b. Children with developmental dysphasia show an abnormal P3b recovery cycle

  c. In contingent negative variation experiments, barbiturates produce positive shifts

  d. In schizophrenia there is generally an increase in the amplitude of P3

  e. P3b may be a marker for conscious thought (SBN)

76. All of the following statements about evoked potentials are true except:

  a. As measured by auditory evoked potentials, cochlear but not brainstem lesions alter early waves

  b. In multiple sclerosis there is a delay in onset of P100

  c. In myoclonic epilepsy there is a low-amplitude evoked action potential

  d. Leukodystrophies produce delayed evoked potentials

  e. The pathological nature of somatosensory evoked potential seen in multiple sclerosis is due to degeneration of axon from the first-order neuron (SBN)

77. All of the following statements about the genetics of personality are true except:

   a. Assortative mating is much greater for personality than for cognitive ability

   b. Functional serotonin transporter polymorphism is associated with neuroticism

   c. Heritabilities in the range 30–50% are typical of personality results

   d. Individuals with longer DRD4 alleles have significantly higher novelty-seeking scores

   e. Openness has less non-additive genetic variance than conscientiousness (PG)

78. Linkage studies have implicated all of the following loci in schizophrenia except:

   a. 1q21-q22

   b. 6p24-22

   c. 6q

   d. 8p22-21

   e. 21q11 (PG)

79. All of the following statements about the genetics of schizophrenia are true except:

   a. T>C polymorphism at nucleotide 102 in the HTR2A gene has been implicated

   b. Homozygosity for Ser9Gly polymorphism in exon 1 of the DRD3 gene has been implicated

   c. Unidentified CAG/CTG repeats are less common in people with schizophrenia than in the general population

   d. Variable findings have been reported with regard to the DRD2 gene that codes for the D_2 receptor

   e. The (1;11) (q42;q14.3) balanced reciprocal translocation generates a LOD score of 3.6 in the schizophrenia phenotype, but of 4.5 in the affective disorders phenotype (PG)

80. Which of the following statements about the genetics of alcohol misuse is true?

    a. The frequency of ADH_2 has been reported to be significantly decreased in members of the Hispanic population with alcoholism

    b. An increased risk of developing alcoholism is associated with the number and proximity of affected relatives

    c. The heritability of alcoholism is 0.25 for males, compared with 0.5 for females

    d. The linkage region on chromosome 11 associated with alcohol misuse is close to the gene that encodes for β_1 GABA

    e. A protective locus has been found on the chromosome t that codes for aldehyde dehydrogenase (PG)

81. All of the following statements about alcohol misuse are true except:

    a. The A1 allele of Taq1 polymorphism close to the DRD_2 gene is associated with alcohol dependence

    b. The ALDH2 responsible for acetaldehyde oxidation maps to chromosome 12q24.2

    c. At intoxicating levels, ADH4 may account for up to 40% of ethanol oxidation

    d. Cytochrome P450IIEI is inhibited by ethanol consumption

    e. The $GABA_A\beta_2$ gene on chromosome 2 has been implicated in alcohol dependence (PG)

82. The following genes have been implicated in the opiate response in mouse models. All of them have been correctly matched except for:

a. DAT – increased reward response

b. GluR-A – reduced tolerance

c. Mu opioid – physical dependence

d. Nociceptin receptor – loss of tolerance

e. SubP – increase in withdrawal (PG)

83. Which of the following is a weak agonist at the μ-receptor?

a. Fentanyl

b. Meperidine

c. Methadone

d. Morphine

e. Buprenorphine (N)

84. Which of the following is a drug that shows agonist activity at the μ-receptor and antagonist activity at the κ-receptor?

a. Buprenorphine

b. Nalorphine

c. Naltrexone

d. Naloxone

e. Pentazocine (N)

85. Which of the following is a drug that shows agonist activity at the δ- and κ-receptors and antagonistic activity at the μ-receptor?

a. Buprenorphine

b. Nalorphine

c. Naltrexone

d. Naloxone

e. Pentazocine (N)

86. Which of the following statements about opioid receptors and endogenous ligands is true?

a. β-endorphin is equipotent on all three types of opioid receptors

b. δ-receptors are supraspinal in distribution

c. Dynorphin is least potent at the κ-receptor

d. Enkephalins are most potent at the κ-receptor

e. Spinal receptors are exclusively of the μ type (N)

87. Which of the following is an antagonist at all three types of opioid receptors?

a. Buprenorphine

b. Fentanyl

c. Nalorphine

d. Naltrexone

e. Pentazocine (N)

88. On which of the following chromosomes is the APP gene located?

a. 3

b. 10

c. 14

d. 17

e. 21 (PG)

89. On which of the following chromosomes is the presenilin-1 gene located?

    a. 3

    b. 10

    c. 14

    d. 17

    e. 21 (PG)

90. Presenilin is involved in controlling:

    a. α-secretase

    b. β-secretase

    c. γ-secretase

    d. δ-secretase

    e. μ-secretase (PG)

91. The polymorphic form that may be protective against developing dementia is:

    a. ApoE1

    b. ApoE2

    c. ApoE3

    d. ApoE4

    e. ApoE5 (PG)

92. The most common genotype associated with type III hyperlipidaemia is:

    a. ApoE1

    b. ApoE2

    c. ApoE3

    d. ApoE4

    e. ApoE5 (PG)

93. Which of the following is associated with prolonged QT_c intervals?

  a. Chamomile

  b. Hops

  c. Kava

  d. Passionflower

  e. Valerian (BJP 2006)

94. All of the following statements about the course of affective disorder are true except:

  a. Agoraphobia without panic disorder lacks evidence for influencing course

  b. Anxiety disorders present during relative euthymia predict a worse prognosis

  c. Current comorbid anxiety disorder is associated with a risk of earlier relapse

  d. A longer time period since the resolution of a previous episode predicts subsyndromal symptoms in recurrent unipolar depression

  e. Social anxiety disorder is associated with poor outcomes of bipolar disorder (BJP 2006)

95. Which of the following statements about crisis resolution/home treatment teams (CRHTs) is true?

  a. Adding assertive outreach teams to existing services did not produce a significant change in hospital admissions

  b. CRHTs significantly reduce the admission of younger adults

  c. Changes in admission patterns are not sustained for 3 months following the setting up of CRHTs

  d. CHRTs cause a significant reduction in the number of admissions of older men

  e. None of the above (BJP 2006)

96. Which of the following statements about benzodiazepine discontinuation is true?

    a. Around 1% of the general population uses benzodiazepines

    b. The augmentation of systematic discontinuation with group CBT is no more effective than systematic discontinuation alone

    c. The augmentation of systematic discontinuation with carbamazepine is more effective than systematic discontinuation alone

    d. The odds ratio for minimal intervention is 2.8 compared with treatment as usual

    e. Systematic discontinuation programmes are significantly more effective than simple advice (BJP 2006)

97. All of the following statements about debriefing are true except:

    a. Debriefing in people with high baseline levels of arousal increases their likelihood of developing PTSD

    b. Emotional ventilation debriefing is safer than educational debriefing

    c. Psychoeducation provided as part of debriefing may increase awareness of stress symptoms

    d. There is no empirical evidence to support single-session debriefing for anxiety

    e. There is evidence for adverse effects of debriefing for PTSD (BJP 2006)

98. All of the following statements about schizophrenia are true except:

a. Group II metabotropic glutamate-receptor antagonists show antipsychotic efficacy

b. Group II metabotropic receptors are autoreceptors that inhibit glutamate release

c. Lexical verbal fluency is less impaired with schizophrenia than is semantic verbal fluency

d. Schizophrenia involves an increased speed of activation in semantic memory

e. Semantic verbal fluency may be the best candidate for cognitive endophenotype (BJP 2008)

99. All of the following statements about affective disorders are true except:

a. Family therapy is neither more nor less effective than crisis management for bipolar disorder

b. Group psychoeducation as an adjunct to pharmacological therapy may be effective for relapse prevention in bipolar disorder

c. Internet-delivered brief CBT may be effective in the treatment of depression

d. Male gender and depression are associated with self-harm in first-episode psychosis

e. Progressive severity of depressive episodes is dependent on the patient's age at the onset of the disorder (BJP 2008)

100. Which of the following statements about eating disorders is true?

    a. Women with anorexia are more likely to experience preterm birth than women with bulimia

    b. The lifetime risk of bulimia nervosa in adult women is 3%

    c. The rate of partial syndrome in eating disorder is less than that of anorexia nervosa

    d. Women with anorexia nervosa are more likely to deliver babies of normal birth weight than those in the general population

    e. Women with bulimia have significantly higher rates of past miscarriages than those in the general population (BJP 2007 and 2008)

101. All of the following statements about the genetics of schizophrenia are true except:

    a. Delta-9-tetrahydrocannabinol acts through the CNR1 receptor

    b. CHRNA7 variation alters the risk of schizophrenia

    c. Higher than normal levels of glutamine are found in the anterior cingulate of never-treated patients

    d. Paternal age is consistently associated with the risk of schizophrenia

    e. Tobacco alleviates neurophysiological deficits through activity at the α_7-nicotinic cholinergic receptor (BJP 2007)

102. Which of the following statements about early psychosis is true?

    a. The 3-year prevalence of adolescent-onset schizophrenia is 3 per 100 000 in the general population

    b. Impaired emotional recognition is not seen among the healthy siblings of patients with schizophrenia

    c. Later childhood growth is associated with schizophrenia spectrum disorder

    d. There is an association between relatively slow early growth and schizophrenia in women

    e. There is no association between a lack of insight and the stability of substance-induced psychosis diagnosis (BJP 2007)

103. Urea can be measured by using:

    a. ^{19}F

    b. ^{1}h

    c. ^{2}h

    d. ^{14}N

    e. ^{31}P (KS)

104. pO_2 can be measured by using:

    a. ^{19}F

    b. ^{1}H

    c. ^{2}H

    d. ^{14}N

    e. ^{31}P (KS)

105. pH can be measured by using:

    a. ^{19}F

    b. ^{1}H

    c. ^{2}H

    d. ^{14}N

    e. ^{31}P (KS)

106. The rCBF technique involves:

    a. Fluorine-18

    b. Iodine-123

    c. Nitrogen-13

    d. Technetium-99 m

    e. Xenon-133 (KS)

107. Blood flow is measured by using:

    a. Fluorine-18

    b. l-hexamethyl-propylene amine oxime

    c. Iodine-123

    d. Nitrogen-13

    e. Xenon-133 (KS)

108. Renal calculi are an adverse effect of:

    a. Gabapentin

    b. Levitracetam

    c. Pregabalin

    d. Tiagabine

    e. Topiramate (KS)

109. Which of the following statements about paraldehyde is true?

   a. It blocks the sedating effects of alcohol

   b. Disulfiram increases the metabolism of paraldehyde

   c. An overdose leads to respiratory acidosis

   d. The unmetabolised drug is expired by the lungs

   e. It has a wide therapeutic range (KS)

110. Gaboxadol acts at which of the following α-subunits of the GABA receptor?

   a. 1

   b. 2

   c. 3

   d. 4

   e. 5 (KS)

111. All of the following statements about flumazenil are true except:

   a. It can reverse the effects of zaleplon

   b. It can precipitate seizures

   c. It does not reverse the effects of opioids

   d. It should be used only once at a dosage of 2 mg

   e. Sedation can return in up to 3% of people who are treated with flumazenil (KS)

112. All of the following are interactions of bupropion except:

   a. Carbamazepine – increases the concentration of bupropion

   b. Levodopa – delirium

   c. Lithium – CNS toxicity

   d. MAOIs – hypertensive crisis

   e. Metoprolol – sinus bradycardia (KS)

113. All of the following statements about executive function and stroke are true except:

a. Antidepressants foster long-term but not short-term improvement in executive function after a stroke

b. Antidepressants improve outcome after a stroke which is dependent on the improvement of depression

c. Nortriptyline improves the activities of daily living

d. Antidepressants reorganise brain circuitry by their effect on brain-derived neurotrophic factor

e. Sertraline improves morbidity (BJP 2007)

114. Which of the following statements about frontal-release signs is true?

a. In patients with schizophrenia, frontal-release sign scores show an inverse correlation with IQ

b. In patients with schizophrenia, right-grasp reflex scores correlate negatively with the number of perseverative errors on the Wisconsin Card Sorting Test

c. Single sign scores correlate with clinical pathology

d. They do not occur in healthy young people

e. Strong evidence exists for the heritability of neurological soft signs (BJP 2007)

115. All of the following statements about lithium are true except:

a. About 50% of patients with bipolar disorder are prescribed lithium

b. Glomerular dysfunction is more common than tubular dysfunction

c. It reduces the lethality of suicide attempts

d. It is retained in monotherapy for much longer than other mood stabilisers

e. Treatment adherence is a strong predictor of suicidal behaviour (KS)

116. Which of the following statements about psychotherapy is true?

    a. Brief CBT influences long-term outcomes in patients with acute PTSD

    b. E-CBT reduces the symptom burden of people with social phobia

    c. Integrated therapy for patients with bipolar disorder and substance misuse is no more effective than group drug counselling

    d. Psychoeducation may be as beneficial as CBT in the prevention of relapses of bipolar disorder

    e. There is level A evidence for debriefing as a treatment of post-traumatic stress disorder (BJP 2008)

117. Which of the following genes has been linked to depression?

    a. 4q

    b. 9p

    c. 15q

    d. 18p

    e. 22p (PG)

118. Which of the following statements about the epidemiology of affective disorders is true?

    a. Bipolar type 1 disorder is more common among married men than others

    b. A higher than average incidence of bipolar type 1 disorder is found among people in lower socio-economic groups

    c. The lifetime incidence of OCD is twice as high among patients with major depression as it is among those with bipolar type 1 disorder

    d. The mean age of onset of bipolar type 1 disorder is 30 years

    e. The mean age of onset of depression is 20 years (KS)

119. All of the following statements about the role of amines in affect-ive disorders are true except:

    a. Cholinergic agonists can exacerbate the symptoms of depression

    b. A correlation exists between the down-regulation of β-adrenergic receptors and the clinical antidepressant response

    c. The D_1-receptor may be hypoactive in depression

    d. GABA-receptors are upregulated by antidepressants

    e. The platelets of people with suicidal impulses have a high concentration of serotonin uptake sites (KS)

120. Which of the following statements about the neuroendocrine pathology of affective disorders is true?

    a. The gene coding for neurokinin-mediated BDNF increases after chronic stress

    b. Hypercortisolaemia in depression suggests increased activity from acetylcholine

    c. Increased CSF somatostatin levels have been reported in depression

    d. In affective disorders there is increased feedback inhibition from the hippocampus over the hypothalamo–pituitary–adrenal axis

    e. Around 10% of depressed individuals show a blunted TSH response to a TRH challenge (KS)

121. Which of the following patient variables is necessary for psy-chodynamic psychotherapy?

    a. The ability to modulate regression

    b. A modest to moderate need for direction and guidance

    c. Responsiveness to behavioural thinking

    d. Responsiveness to environmental manipulation

    e. Social or communication problems (KS)

122. All of the following are limitations of psychodynamic theory except:

    a. Enduring structural change transcends symptomatic relief

    b. Its focus on intrapsychic phenomena may obscure other factors

    c. Long-term open-ended treatment is uneconomical

    d. Personality alteration can be too ambitious

    e. Transference regression can lead to over-idealisation of the therapist (KS)

123. All of the following are indications for pharmacotherapy in depression except:

    a. Depressive stupor

    b. Early-morning wakening

    c. Loss of control over thinking

    d. Low self-esteem

    e. Marked vegetative signs (KS)

124. All of the following statements about phototherapy are true except:

    a. It is well tolerated

    b. The light range that it uses is between 500 and 1000 lux

    c. Longer treatment durations are associated with better responses

    d. Sleep disorders in geriatric patients can improve with bright light during the day

    e. It is used between 1 and 2 hours before dawn (KS)

125. With which of the following is priapism seen?

    a. Duloxetine

    b. Maprotiline

    c. Nefazadone

    d. Trazadone

    e. Trimipramine (KS)

126. The hallmark of which of the following therapies is its patients' ability to be their true selves in the face of familial or other pressures that threaten them with the loss of social position or love?

    a. The Bowen model

    b. The general systems model

    c. The psychodynamic–experiential model

    d. The social network model

    e. The structural model (KS)

127. In which of the following is the patient encouraged to engage in unwanted behaviour?

    a. The Bowen model

    b. Conjoint therapy

    c. The general systems model

    d. Paradoxical therapy

    e. Reframing (KS)

128. The most common form of marital therapy is:

    a. Combined therapy

    b. Conjoint therapy

    c. Four-way session

    d. Individual therapy

    e. Individual couple therapy (KS)

129. The form of couples therapy in which a different therapist sees each partner, with regular joint sessions in which all of the participants take part, is called:

    a. Combined therapy

    b. Conjoint therapy

    c. Four-way session

    d. Individual therapy

    e. Individual couple therapy (KS)

130. The modes of treatment in DBT include all of the following except:

    a. Consultation team

    b. Group skills training

    c. Individual therapy

    d. Telephone consultation

    e. Termination letter (KS)

Paper 4

1. With regard to the treatment of premenstrual syndrome, all of the following statements are false except:

   a. Danazol worsens mastalgia

   b. Dosing in the luteal phase is less efficacious than treatment throughout the cycle

   c. Fluoxetine is safer than other treatments, as it does not alter the length of the menstrual cycle

   d. SSRIs are efficacious in treating both physiological and psychological symptoms

   e. The onset of improvement following SSRI treatment is much slower than with depressive disorder (APT 2007)

2. All of the following statements about the withdrawal symptoms seen in neonates due to maternal use of antidepressants are true except:

   a. They are associated with maternal SSRI use in late pregnancy

   b. They are associated with maternal use of tricyclic antidepressants in late gestation

   c. Such symptoms are absent at birth

   d. Such symptoms include tremor and feeding difficulties

   e. Such symptoms usually resolve within 2 weeks (APT 2007)

3. All of the following statements about the Clinical Antipsychotic Trials of Intervention Effectiveness (CATIE) are true except:

   a. The Brief Psychiatric Rating Scale was their measure of primary outcome

   b. They involved double-blind randomised trials

   c. The duration of the study was 18 months

   d. Patients with tardive dyskinesia were excluded from the perphenazine arm

   e. Their proxy for effectiveness was the discontinuation of treatment for any cause (APT 2008)

4. All of the following were outcomes from the CATIE except:

   a. Discontinuation due to intolerable side-effects was greatest with olanzapine

   b. The initial large improvement from olanzapine was not sustained by the end of the study

   c. Olanzapine treatment was less costly than treatment with perphenazine

   d. The overall rate of discontinuation of the antipsychotics was 74%

   e. There was no significant difference between the drugs with regard to the incidence of extrapyramidal side-effects (APT 2008)

5. All of the following were features of the Cost Utility of the Latest Antipsychotic Drugs in Schizophrenia Study (CUtLASS) except:

   a. The clinicians used haloperidol infrequently

   b. The patients on second-generation antipsychotics showed a trend towards greater improvement in terms of quality of life than others

   c. It was a multi-centre trial

   d. It found no clear patient preference with regard to choice of antipsychotics

   e. Its specific hypothesis was that new antipsychotics would be associated with a clinically significant improvement in quality of life for 1 year over that of older drugs (APT 2008)

6. Mr Allen is to be started on an atypical antipsychotic. He knows that his father suffered from parkinsonism due to having been on a typical antipsychotic. He would like to know what the predisposing factors are for atypical antipsychotic drug-induced parkinsonism. All of the following are predisposing factors except:

   a. A higher than BNF maximum dose

   b. A higher starting dose

   c. Being male

   d. Increasing age

   e. An individual predisposition to a high rate of dopaminergic neuron loss (APT 2008)

7. Mr Redbridge has a diagnosis of chronic schizophrenia. You suspect that he has negative symptoms, whilst the neurologist's opinion is that he has parkinsonian features. All of the following factors support your diagnosis except:

a. Avoidance of eye contact

b. Loss of intonation of speech

c. Preserved articulation of speech

d. Preserved spontaneous generation of words

e. Restricted range and depth of mood (APT 2008)

8. All of the following statements about EEG monitoring of ECT are true except:

a. A study conducted in India found that 10–15% of its sample had prolonged seizures on EEG

b. The end point is the most likely point at which the immediate post-ictal tracing begins

c. The incidence of prolonged ECT was 1% in the Edinburgh ECT clinic

d. The potential clinical application of ictal EEG does not include a prediction of eventual treatment response

e. There is a lack of significant correlation between post-ictal suppression and clinical improvement (APT 2007)

9. To which of the following is the quality of ictal EEG significantly related?

a. Age

b. Concurrent medications

c. Electrode placement

d. Previous ECT episodes

e. Threshold dose (APT 2007)

10. All of the following statements about ethnicity and psychiatric disorders in the UK are true except:

    a. The EMPIRIC report showed that higher rates of Pakistani women reported common mental disorders compared with the general population

    b. The EMPIRIC report showed that lower rates of Bangladeshi women reported common mental disorders compared with the general population

    c. The EMPIRIC report showed that there was twice as much psychotic illness in people of African and Caribbean origin compared with the general population

    d. People of African and Caribbean origin are more likely to be detained against their will

    e. Young people of African-Caribbean origin continue to be at five times less risk of suicide and self-harm than white British people (APT 2008)

11. For which of the following herbal remedies does evidence exist for its effectiveness in treating anxiety?

    a. *Ginkgo biloba*

    b. *Lavandula angustifolia*

    c. *Melissa officinalis*

    d. *Piper methysticum*

    e. *Valeriana officinalis* (APT 2007)

12. Which of the following has been shown to be an ineffective remedy for treating depression?

    a. *Crocus sativus*

    b. *Ginkgo biloba*

    c. *Hypericum perforatum*

    d. *Lavandula angustifolia*

    e. All of the above (APT 2007)

13. Which of the following statements about the epidemiology of medically unexplained psychological symptoms is true?

    a. Around 5–10% of all primary care consultations are for medically unexplained psychological symptoms

    b. Less than 25% of patients who have debilitating fatigue lasting more than 6 months also have fibromyalgia

    c. 'Medically unexplained symptom' is the term preferred by GPs

    d. Most patients with medically unexplained symptoms do not allow their doctors an opportunity to address their psychological needs

    e. The number of such symptoms over a person's lifetime shows a linear correlation with the number of anxiety but not depressive disorders the person has experienced (APT 2008)

14. Which of the following statements about the aetiological understanding of medically unexplained symptoms is true?

    a. Children of parents with medically unexplained symptoms are at lower risk of such a presentation than the children of parents with organic conditions

    b. Children with higher academic competence show a higher rate of medically unexplained symptoms

    c. GPs tend to have the attitude that such symptoms should be managed in primary care

    d. Intergenerational transmission is understood purely as social learning

    e. Physical and emotional, but not sexual, abuse in childhood is related to such symptoms (APT 2008)

15. Which of the following statements about the treatment of medically unexplained psychological symptoms is true?

    a. The benefits from antidepressant treatment are dependent on the presence of depression

    b. No treatment has been demonstrated to be effective in secondary care

    c. One session of psychological therapy may reduce the number of GP visits

    d. A somatic symptom that lasts for more than 1 year is indicative of a poor prognosis

    e. The reattribution model of treatment has five stages (APT 2008)

16. With which of the following are passivity phenomena associated?

    a. Hypoactivation of the right inferior parietal cortex

    b. Hypoactivation of the right parietal cortex

    c. Hyperactivation of the supplementary motor area

    d. Reduced grey matter in the dominant parietal lobe

    e. Reduced grey matter in the non-dominant prefrontal cortex (APT 2006)

17. Which of the following statements about abnormal bodily perceptions and delusions is true?

    a. Somatic hallucinations activate the primary somatosensory and posterior parietal cortex

    b. Body dysmorphic disorder is associated with abnormal putamen circuits

    c. Conversion disorder with motor symptoms is associated with inhibition of the orbitofrontal cortex

    d. They involve hyperperfusion of the left temporo-parietal cortex

    e. Reduced striatal D_2-receptor binding occurs in Cotard's syndrome (APT 2006)

18. All of the following observations about self-harm are true except:

   a. Around 40% of the people who attend A&E following self-harm have taken an overdose

   b. Cutting may be twice as prevalent as overdosing in community samples

   c. The majority of the people who self-injure do not go to a hospital

   d. One important factor in not seeking hospital treatment is a previous poor experience in A&E

   e. One quarter of all suicides are preceded by self-harm episodes during the year before they occur (APT 2007)

19. Which of the following observations about self-injury is true?

   a. Among young adults, significantly more females use self-injury to kill themselves than do males

   b. In a household survey, 5% of the men who were surveyed admitted to self-harm without suicidal intent

   c. People who present with cutting are less likely to present with suicidal intent than people who present with self-poisoning

   d. Repeated self-injury is associated with sexual abuse in women but not in men

   e. The UK has one of the highest incidences of self-injury among schoolchildren of any country (APT 2006)

20. All of the following observations about self-injury are true except:

    a. Among children and adolescents, females are more likely than males to say that they have to tried to obtain relief from an unbearable state of mind

    b. Individuals who present with self-cutting behaviour have reported feeling less pain than matched controls

    c. Individuals who poison themselves are more impulsive than those who cut themselves

    d. In females, body shame is positively correlated with self-harming behaviour

    e. Self-poisoning is a strong predictor of suicide in people with schizophrenia (APT 2006)

21. Which of the following statements about the treatment strategy for self-injury is true?

    a. Manual-assisted CBT is a cost-effective method for reducing self-harming behaviour in patients with borderline personality disorder

    b. Naltrexone at a dose of 50 mg/day can reduce self-harming behaviour when other measures have failed

    c. Self-harming behaviour in borderline personality disorder with dissociative states has been shown to benefit little from dialectical behaviour therapy in secure units

    d. Significant evidence suggests that people grow out of self-harming behaviour

    e. Evidence exists which suggests that safety agreements between staff and patients reduce self-harming behaviour (APT 2006)

22. All of the following statements about smoking are true except:

    a. Approximately 50% of smokers with mental illness in the UK have shown a desire to quit smoking

    b. High rates of smoking are significantly associated with an increased risk of other smoking-related illnesses in people with mental illness

    c. People whose mental illness has remitted are at no greater risk of subsequent smoking than people with active disorders

    d. People with mental illness are three times more likely to smoke than the general population

    e. Smoking increases the risk of mental illness even after correcting for major risk indicators of a mental disorder (APT 2008)

23. EEG in subacute sclerosing panencephalitis shows:

    a. Irregular theta activity

    b. Low-voltage EEG

    c. Triphasic waves

    d. Periodic complex

    e. 3 Hz spike and wave (SBN)

24. With which of the following changes in EEG are negative symptoms in schizophrenia correlated?

    a. Decreased alpha activity

    b. Increased beta activity

    c. Increased delta wave

    d. Low mean alpha frequency

    e. Paroxysmal activity (SBN)

25. Which of the following does EEG of autistic spectrum disorders show?

    a. Alpha deficits

    b. Beta deficits

    c. Beta excess

    d. Delta excess

    e. Theta excess (SBN)

26. All of the following are characteristics of alpha waves except:

    a. They are measured at 8 to 12 Hz

    b. They are attenuated with attention

    c. They are bilateral and frontal

    d. They have a higher amplitude on the dominant side

    e. They are seen in a relaxed state with the eyes closed (SBN)

27. A generalised epileptiform pattern of EEG is seen with:

    a. Alcohol

    b. Benzodiazepine

    c. Cannabis

    d. Cocaine

    e. Phencyclidine (SBN)

28. The shoulder is supplied by:

    a. C3

    b. C4

    c. C5

    d. C6

    e. C7 (TN)

29. With which of the following are the Ib fibres associated?

   a. Pressure

   b. Primary sensory output from muscle spindles

   c. Secondary sensory terminals of muscle spindles

   d. Sensory fibres of Golgi tendon organs

   e. Touch (TN)

30. With which of the following fibre types does the fusimotor to intrafusal fibres of muscle spindles function match?

   a. Aβ afferent

   b. Aδ afferent

   c. C afferent

   d. Aα efferent

   e. Aγ efferent (TN)

31. In which of the following are contralateral pain and temperature sensation loss with ipsilateral weakness and loss of proprioception seen?

   a. Brown–Sequard syndrome

   b. Ependymoma

   c. Syringomyelia

   d. Tabes dorsalis

   e. Spina bifida (TN)

32. In which of the following are the gyri of Heschl?

   a. Broca's area

   b. The primary auditory cortex

   c. The primary motor area

   d. The primary somaesthetic area

   e. Wernicke's area (TN)

33. Which of the following statements about the anterolateral system is true?

    a. It is involved in the transmission of discriminative touch

    b. Its first-order neurons are bipolar

    c. Unmyelinated C fibres in the pain pathway transmit sensations that elicit an affective response

    d. Around 15% of its nociceptive fibres project to the thalamus via a relay in the reticular formation

    e. The spinothalamic tract sends inputs to the dorsolateral nucleus of the thalamus (TN)

34. All of the following statements about the vibration sense are true except:

    a. Decussation is in the medial lemniscus

    b. The cell bodies of first-order neurons are located in the dorsal root ganglion

    c. The cell bodies of second-order neurons are located in the dorsal horn

    d. The VPL nucleus of the thalamus hosts the cell bodies of third-order neurons

    e. Third-order neurons terminate in the postcentral gyrus (TN)

35. Which of the following statements about the ascending sensory tracts to the cerebellum is true?

    a. The anterior cerebellar tract terminates in the ipsilateral anterior lobe of the cerebellum

    b. The cell bodies of first-order neurons are located in the dorsal root ganglion

    c. Second-order neuron cell bodies belonging to the cuneocerebellar tract are located in the dorsal horn

    d. Most of the proprioception information reaches conscious levels

    e. The rostral spinocerebellar tract coordinates the movements of the lower limb muscles (TN)

36. Mr Bainbridge presents with muscle weakness, loss of vibratory sense, two-point discrimination and proprioception. This is due to:

    a. Brown–Sequard syndrome

    b. Friedrich's ataxia

    c. Subacute combined degeneration

    d. Syringomyelia

    e. Tabes dorsalis (TN)

37. Mr Bainbridge presents with loss of pain and temperature sensation from the skin of both shoulders and upper extremities, followed by weakness and atrophy of the intrinsic muscles of the hand. This is due to:

    a. Brown–Sequard syndrome

    b. Friedrich's ataxia

    c. Subacute combined degeneration

    d. Syringomyelia

    e. Tabes dorsalis (TN)

38. Which of the following are the afferent fibres that pass through the inferior cerebellar peduncle?

   a. The anterior spinocerebellar tract

   b. The ceruleocerebellar fibres

   c. The rubrocerebellar fibres

   d. The tectocerebellar fibres

   e. The trigeminocerebellar fibres (TN)

39. From which of the following do the monoaminergic fibres that terminate only in the granular and molecular layers of the cerebellar cortex originate?

   a. The deep cerebellar nuclei

   b. The hypothalamus

   c. The locus coeruleus

   d. The pontine raphe nuclei

   e. The ventral midbrain tegmentum (TN)

40. Mr Bainbridge presents with an inability to maintain equilibrium. An examination reveals no evidence of ataxia, hypotonia or tremor. He tends to sway from side to side when he walks. The examination also reveals nystagmus. To which of the following is this probably due?

   a. Flocculonodular syndrome

   b. Left hemispheric zone disorder

   c. Paravermal zone disorder

   d. Vermal zone disorder

   e. Right hemispheric zone disorder (TN)

41. With which of the following cranial nerves is the pterygopalatine ganglion associated?

    a. III

    b. V

    c. VII

    d. IX

    e. X (TN)

42. The sensory ganglion belonging to the trigeminal nerve is the:

    a. Ciliary

    b. Geniculate

    c. Gasserian

    d. Scarpa's

    e. Submandibular (TN)

43. Which of the following nuclei regulates the release of reproductive hormones from the adenohypophysis?

    a. Arcuate

    b. Lateral preoptic

    c. Periventricular

    d. Preoptic

    e. Supraoptic (TN)

44. Which of the following is the body's master clock?

    a. Arcuate

    b. Mamillary

    c. Medial preoptic

    d. Supraoptic

    e. Suprachiasmatic (TN)

45. Which of the following is the thalamic nucleus involved in learning and memory?

a. The anterior

b. The dorsal midline

c. The ventral midline

d. The pulvinar

e. The parvocellular (TN)

46. In which of the following is the medial geniculate body involved?

a. Hearing

b. The integration of somatosensory information

c. Sensorimotor integration

d. Taste

e. Vision (TN)

47. Mr Bainbridge presents with allodynia, hyperpathia and dysesthesia. To which of the following is this due?

a. Brown–Sequard syndrome

b. Dejerine–Roussy syndrome

c. Guillain–Barré syndrome

d. Kluver–Bucy syndrome

e. Stevens–Johnson syndrome (TN)

48. Which of the following is a feature of a right-hemisphere lesion?

a. Acalculia

b. Alexia without agraphia

c. Broca's aphasia

d. Colour anomia without agraphia

e. Prosopagnosia (SBN)

49. All of the following are features of a left-hemisphere lesion except:

a. Agraphia without alexia

b. Alexia with agraphia

c. Constructional apraxia

d. Gerstmann's syndrome

e. Wernicke's aphasia (SBN)

50. All of the following statements about hypothalamic connections are true except that they go:

a. To the amygdala via the amygdalofugal bundle

b. To the amygdala via the stria terminalis

c. To the anterior thalamus via the mammillothalamic tract

d. To the hippocampus via the fornix

e. To the septum via the lateral forebrain bundle (SBN)

51. Which of the following statements about the anatomy of the limbic system is true?

a. The amygdala lies in the medial aspect of the frontal lobe

b. The limbic system controls the autonomic nervous system via the medial longitudinal fasciculus

c. Major output from the mammillary bodies flows to the posterior nucleus of the thalamus

d. The mammillary bodies receive a number of axons through the stria terminalis

e. The septal nuclei have reciprocal connections with the hippocampus via the fornix (SBN)

52. Which of the following statements about the arousal system is true?

   a. The cholinergic pathways are independent of the arousal system

   b. During relaxed wakefulness, descending reticulospinal projections increase the sensitivity of the stretch reflex arcs

   c. Projections from the reticular nuclei of the thalamus produce a characteristic beta-wave form on an EEG

   d. The reticular formation in the midbrain surrounds the aqueduct of Sylvius

   e. The reticular formation projects to the ventroposterolateral nucleus of the thalamus (SBN)

53. Which of the following statements about serotonergic receptors is true?

   a. $5-HT_{1A}$ receptors are found in raphe cell bodies

   b. $5-HT_{1c}$ is found in the heart

   c. β-Blockers are agonists at $5-HT_{1B}$

   d. LSD is an agonist at $5-HT_3$

   e. Ritanserin is an agonist at $5-HT_{2A}$ (SBN)

54. Which of the following statements about serotonin is true?

   a. Decreasing concentration produces bizarre stereotyped behaviour

   b. High CSF 5-HIAA predicts impulsivity

   c. Increasing concentrations lead to insomnia

   d. The postsynaptic $5-HT_1$ receptor mediating prolactin release is blunted in depression

   e. Selective uptake blockers cause weight gain (SBN)

55. Which of the following statements about opioid receptors is true?

   a. β-Endorphin is an antagonist at the μ-receptor

   b. Enkephalins are endogenous agonists of the δ-receptor

   c. Naloxone is an agonist at the μ-receptor

   d. Naltrexone is an agonist at the μ-receptor

   e. Pentazocine is an antagonist at the κ-receptor (SBN)

56. All of the following statements about peptides are true except:

   a. CCK_A is involved in emotional behaviour

   b. CRH stimulates locus firing

   c. Injections of CRH produce decreased appetite

   d. TRH is three amino acids long

   e. Two different types of CCK receptors have been identified (SBN)

57. Non-urgent CT is indicated in all of the following except:

   a. Encephalitis

   b. Confusion for which no metabolic or toxic cause has been found

   c. Marked and persistent or variable drowsiness

   d. Schizophrenia developing after the age of 40 years

   e. Progressive cognitive decline developing after the age of 65 years (SBN)

58. Mr Bainbridge is a 60-year-old man. He presents with a bitemporal headache which he describes as being a pressure-like pain. He has had a history of migraine and is on medications. The most plausible diagnosis is:

a. Cluster headache

b. Cranial arteritis

c. Malignant hypertension

d. Migraine

e. Tension headache (SBN)

59. Mr Bainbridge presents with a headache on waking which seems to improve with a change of posture. The diagnosis is:

a. Arteriovenous malformations

b. Cluster headache

c. Hypertensive encephalopathy

d. Obstructive hydrocephalus

e. Temporal arteritis (SBN)

60. Mr Bainbridge presents with an occipital headache, vertigo, diplopia, blurring of vision and lethargy. The diagnosis is:

a. Cluster headache

b. Cranial arteritis

c. Hypertensive encephalopathy

d. Migraine

e. A space-occupying lesion (SBN)

61. An EEG shows a 2/s spike and wave form in a person with a clinical history of absences. The diagnosis is:

    a. Benign rolandic epilepsy

    b. Creutzfeldt–Jacob disease

    c. Huntington's disease

    d. Lennox–Gastaut syndrome

    e. Temporal-lobe epilepsy (SBN)

62. All of the following statements about blepharospasm are true except:

    a. It is associated with demyelinating disorders

    b. It is more common in men than in women

    c. l-DOPA can cause blepharospasm

    d. Spontaneous remission occurs in only 10% of patients

    e. Its symptom presents bilaterally (SBN)

63. All of the following tests form a part of the Halstead–Reitan Battery except:

    a. The Aphasia Screen

    b. The Seashore Rhythm Test

    c. The Stroop Colour–Word Interference Test

    d. The Tactual Performance Test

    e. The Wechsler Adult Intelligence Scale (Revised) (SBN)

64. All of the following are clinical scales of the Standardised Luria–Nebraska Battery except:

    a. Expressive speech

    b. Motor

    c. Power

    d. Receptive speech

    e. Rhythm (SBN)

65. All of the following statements about the timing of the course of events occurring after an occlusion of a cerebral vessel are true except:

    a. Less than 12 hours – no microscopic or macroscopic changes by conventional methods

    b. 12 to 24 hours – increasing swelling of damaged area with normal staining of the brain

    c. 1 to 3 days – inflammatory cell response

    d. 1 to 2 weeks – astrocytosis

    e. Months or years – tissue destruction with remaining astrocytic scar or cavity formation (SBN)

66. All of the following statements about intracranial haemorrhages are true except:

    a. Extradural haemorrhages are commonly due to a laceration of the middle meningeal artery

    b. Lacunar disease presents more commonly in relation to basal ganglia when it involves grey matter

    c. Oral contraception increases the risk of a subarachnoid haemorrhage

    d. Subacute subdural haematomas are due to the rupturing of the veins that join the superior sagittal sinus

    e. The most common cause of subarachnoid haemorrhages is an extension from a bleed elsewhere within the cranium (SBN)

67. The most common cause of acute bacterial meningitis in people of any age is:

    a. *E. coli*

    b. *Haemophilus influenzae*

    c. *Neisseria meningitidis*

    d. *Staphylococcus aureus*

    e. *Streptococcus pneumoniae* (SBN)

68. In the intermediate lobe of the pituitary, all of the following are derived from pro-opiomelanocortin except:

  a. α-Melanocyte-stimulating hormone

  b. Adrenocorticotrophic hormone

  c. β-Endorphin

  d. γ-Lipotrophin

  e. Corticotrophin-like intermediate lobe peptide (SBN)

69. Guanylate cyclase is activated by:

  a. ACTH

  b. Adenosine

  c. Angiotensin II

  d. Arginine vasopressin

  e. Atrial natriuretic peptide (SBN)

70. Adenylyl cyclase is inhibited by:

  a. ACTH

  b. Adenosine

  c. Angiotensin II

  d. Arginine vasopressin

  e. Atrial natriuretic peptide (SBN)

71. Adenylyl cyclase is activated by all of the following except:

  a. Calcitonin

  b. Follicle-stimulating hormone

  c. Glucagon

  d. Insulin

  e. Thyroid-stimulating hormone (SBN)

72. Phosphoinositide turnover is controlled by:

a. Glucagon

b. Histamine

c. Human chorionic gonadotropin

d. Insulin

e. Thyrotropin-releasing hormone (SBN)

73. All of the following statements about the genetics of cognitive abilities are true except:

a. An allele of APOE is associated with cognitive decline in an unselected population of elderly men

b. Differences in the number of fragile X sequences in the normal range are correlated with the differences in 'g'

c. The genes found to be associated with spatial ability are likely to be associated with verbal ability

d. Heterozygotes for phenylketonuria show slightly lowered IQ scores

e. There is no genetic link between severe learning disability and normal variations in IQ (PG)

74. All of the following are autosomal dominant disorders except:

a. Apert syndrome

b. Hurler syndrome

c. Noonan syndrome

d. Treacher–Collins syndrome

e. Tuberous sclerosis (PG)

75. In which of the following conditions does IQ gradually deteriorate after the age of 2 years?

   a. Apert syndrome

   b. Hurler syndrome

   c. Noonan syndrome

   d. Treacher–Collins syndrome

   e. Tuberous sclerosis (PG)

76. In which of the following is aphasia seen?

   a. ATR-X syndrome

   b. Coffin–Lowry syndrome

   c. Fragile X syndrome

   d. Rett syndrome

   e. X-linked hydrocephalus (PG)

77. In which of the following are abnormalities involving MECP2 on Xq28 seen?

   a. ATR-X syndrome

   b. Coffin–Lowry syndrome

   c. Fragile X syndrome

   d. Rett syndrome

   e. X-linked hydrocephalus (PG)

78. Which of the following statements about substance misuse is true?

    a. Family influence predominantly influences maintenance more than initiation

    b. Its heritability is greater for females than for males

    c. Sedative use does not have a heritable component

    d. The Vietnam Era Twin Registry Study reported that heroin shows an effect for non-additive genetics

    e. The Virginia Twin Registry Study strongly implicated family environment for cocaine use in men but not in women (PG)

79. The following genes have been implicated in the cocaine response in mouse models. They have all been correctly matched except for:

    a. 5-HT1B – increased locomotor activity

    b. DRDR1 – increased locomotor activity

    c. GABAA Ab3 – increased locomotor activity

    d. Retinoic acid receptors – blunted response

    e. NAChR beta2 – reduced conditioned place preference (PG)

80. All of the following are ligand-gated ion channels except:

    a. 5-HT_3

    b. $GABA_B$

    c. GluR6

    d. Glycine

    e. nAChR (N)

81. Which of the following statements about the ionic receptor family is true?

    a. Benzodiazepine prolongs the length of time for which the chloride channel is open

    b. The binding site on nAChR is the β-subunit

    c. $GABA_A$ subunits do not share homology with nAChR

    d. The GluR1 subunit of AMPA receptors stimulates the growth of dendritic spines on the cortical pyramidal cells

    e. NMDA receptors favour calcium permeation (N)

82. Which of the following statements about G proteins is true?

    a. Adenylyl cyclase converts cAMP to ATP

    b. GTP binds to the β-subunit

    c. G_s is the second messenger coupled to the $GABA_B$ receptor

    d. G_q activates phospholipase C to cleave PIP_2

    e. Opioid receptors are coupled to the G_q second-messenger system (N)

83. All of the following statements about DNA are true except:

    a. Adenine is always paired with thymine

    b. DNA polymerisation occurs in a 5' to 3' direction

    c. The human genome consists of 3.3×10^9 bases

    d. Transcription involves the formation of RNA from a DNA template

    e. Around 30% of the bases encode proteins (PG)

84. Which of the following statements about the processing of the genetic code is true?

   a. cDNA is the DNA formed from mRNA by the process of reverse transcription

   b. The promoter region is located near the 3′ end of a gene

   c. RNA polymerase I initiates transcription

   d. Splicing involves the removal of exons to produce contiguous mRNA composed only of introns

   e. tRNA has a specific three-base codon sequence (PG)

85. Which of the following statements about the genetic code is true?

   a. AGU is the initiation codon for polypeptide synthesis

   b. All newly synthesised polypeptides start with methionine

   c. An open reading frame is a translation sequence interrupted by a stop codon

   d. UGG is a stop codon

   e. 5′UTR, but not 3′UTR, are not translated (PG)

86. The sequence of DNA that is situated at a defined position on a chromosome is:

   a. An allele

   b. A gene

   c. A locus

   d. mRNA

   e. tRNA (PG)

87. Which of the following statements about mutation is true?

a. Nonsense mutations are also known as silent mutations

b. Non-synonymous substitution results in a change of amino acids

c. The replacement of a DNA sequence with a different one is called an insertion

d. RNA editing involves changing of the nucleotides in RNA before transcription

e. When the allele frequency is less than 0.01, the variants are referred to as mutations (PG)

88. All of the following statements about the 5-HTTLPR gene and depression are true except:

a. The 5-HTTLPR gene has been associated with neuroticism

b. Significant interactions take place between the 5-HTTLPR gene and environmental risk among adolescent women but not adolescent men

c. The 'l' allele increases vulnerability to adverse events

d. The 's' allele reduces the transcriptional efficiency of the serotonin promoter

e. There is no direct relationship between the 5-HTTLPR gene and the onset of depression (BJP 2006)

89. Which of the following statements about adherence therapy is true?

   a. Adherence therapy has a significant advantage over non-specific counselling

   b. Adherence therapy is no more effective than health education for improving quality of life

   c. Adherence rates for prescribed antipsychotic medication are approximately 75%

   d. Clinical interventions for reducing non-adherence are effective in the long term

   e. The relapse rate among a non-adherent sample is twice that of an adherent sample with schizophrenia (BJP 2006)

90. Which of the following statements about inflammatory response and depression is true?

   a. A reduction in CRP occurs following SSRI treatment among patients whose depression resolves, but not among those whose depression remains unresolved

   b. An increased level of CRP is independent of an increased IL-6 concentration

   c. It involves an increased number of neutrophils but not monocytes

   d. Negative acute-phase proteins are increased

   e. SSRIs have an anti-inflammatory effect (BJP 2006)

91. Which of the following statements about manic switch following treatment with antidepressants is true?

    a. Paroxetine has shown a higher switch rate than venlafaxine

    b. The rate of switching to mania or hypomania is greater with bupropion than with desipramine

    c. Switch rates are higher with the newer antidepressants than with tricyclic antidepressants

    d. There is an association between noradrenergic affinity and switch to manic or hypomanic episodes

    e. There is no significant difference between sertraline, venlafaxine and bupropion in causing manic switch (BJP 2006)

92. Which of the following statements about treatment with aripiprazole is true?

    a. It has no effects on the cognitive symptoms of schizophrenia

    b. It may cause more insomnia than typical antipsychotics

    c. It prolongs QT_c intervals more than risperidone does

    d. It is more effective than haloperidol in the treatment of the negative symptoms of schizophrenia

    e. Fewer than 5% of patients who receive this treatment report weight gain (BJP 2006)

93. Which of the following statements about personality disorder and depression is true?

    a. The assessment of personality status early in treatment does not predict the outcome

    b. ECT is associated with poorer outcomes as a treatment for depression that is comorbid with personality disorder than are other therapies

    c. Interpersonal therapy for women with depression and personality disorder is associated with better outcomes than other therapies

    d. The odds ratio for poor outcomes in depressive disorder that is comorbid with personality disorder is 2.18

    e. Significant evidence has been found to suggest that psychotherapy is associated with poor treatment for depression that is comorbid with personality disorder (BJP 2006)

94. Which of the following statements about the neuropathology of schizophrenia is true?

    a. Glial cell densities are reduced when schizophrenia is present

    b. Neuronal density is greater in the left than the right hemisphere when schizophrenia is present

    c. The pyramidal neurons are larger in the left hemisphere when schizophrenia is present

    d. The reversal of asymmetry is most significant in cortical layer 2 when schizophrenia is present

    e. The size and shape of pyramidal neurons do not differ between the two sides in schizophrenia (BJP 2006)

95. Robust evidence has been found for an association between urbanisation and all of the following disorders except:

   a. Anorexia nervosa

   b. Bulimia nervosa

   c. Depression

   d. Psychosis

   e. Schizophrenia (BJP 2006)

96. Which of the following statements about expressed emotion is true?

   a. Critical comments among carers are associated with dependent coping strategies among them

   b. High expressed emotion is an artefact of patient morbidity

   c. A high level of depression in patients is associated with higher levels of expressed emotion among their carers

   d. Hostile but not over-involved family relationships lead to relapses of schizophrenia

   e. Low carer self-esteem is not related to low self-esteem among their patients (BJP 2006)

97. All of the following statements about the treatment of bipolar disorder with eicosapentaenoic acid (EPA) are true except:

   a. A 1 g dose of ethyl-EPA is less effective than a 2 g dose

   b. EPA may inhibit protein kinase C

   c. The incorporation of EPA into cell membranes inhibits the action of phospholipase A_2

   d. More significant improvement is seen on the Hamilton Rating Scale for Depression with adjunctive EPA treatment than with placebo

   e. More significant improvement is seen on adjunctive CGI with EPA than with a placebo (BJP 2006)

98. The triad of optic ataxia, oculomotor apraxia and simultagnosia constitutes:

    a. Apperceptive visual agnosia

    b. Anton's syndrome

    c. Balint's syndrome

    d. Gerstmann's syndrome

    e. Central achromatopsia (KS)

99. Lesions of the dominant parietal lobe cause all of the following except:

    a. Acalculia

    b. Apperceptive visual agnosia

    c. Agraphia

    d. Finger agnosia

    e. Right–left disorientation (KS)

100. All of the following are derived from the telencephalon except the:

    a. Amygdala

    b. Cerebral cortex

    c. Hippocampus

    d. Striatum

    e. Thalamus (KS)

101. All of the following are major anatomical structures involved in semantic memory except the:

    a. Anterior thalamic nuclei

    b. Fornix

    c. Inferolateral temporal lobes

    d. Mammillary body

    e. Prefrontal cortex (KS)

102. All of the following statements about action potentials are true except:

    a. Activation of K^+ channels results in hyperpolarisation

    b. The duration of an action potential in a neuron is 0.1–2 msec

    c. $E_{Cl^-} = -81\,mV$

    d. $E_{Na^+} = 97\,mV$

    e. The spike threshold of a neuron is approximately $-55\,mV$ (KS)

103. Muscarinic receptors can be measured by using:

    a. Fluorine-18

    b. 1-hexamethylpropylene amine oxime

    c. Iodine-123

    d. Nitrogen-13

    e. Xenon-133 (KS)

104. Dopaminergic receptors can be measured by using:

    a. Fluorine-18

    b. 1-hexamethylpropylene amine oxime

    c. Iodine-123

    d. Nitrogen-13

    e. Xenon-133 (KS)

105. A metabolic rate can be measured by using:

    a. Fluorine-18

    b. Oxygen-15

    c. Iodine-123

    d. Nitrogen-13

    e. Xenon-133 (KS)

106. An EEG abnormality seen during caffeine withdrawal is:

   a. Decreased alpha activity

   b. A diffuse slowing of delta waves

   c. Increased beta activity

   d. Increased voltage of theta activity

   e. Non-specific change (KS)

107. An EEG abnormality seen with inhalant use is:

   a. Decreased alpha activity

   b. A diffuse slowing of delta waves

   c. Increased beta activity

   d. Increased voltage of theta activity

   e. Non-specific change (KS)

108. Which of the following statements about the epidemiology of schizophrenia is true?

   a. Its annual incidence is 0.5 to 1.0 per 10 000

   b. The fertility rate for people with schizophrenia is close to that of the general population

   c. The lifetime prevalence of alcoholism within schizophrenia is 25%

   d. Maternal influenza in the third trimester of pregnancy is a risk factor for schizophrenia

   e. Up to 50% of all patients with schizophrenia have significant physical illnesses (KS)

109. All of the following statements about gender differences in schizophrenia are true except:

   a. It is equally prevalent in men and women

   b. Less than half of all male patients but only one-third of all female patients are admitted to a psychiatric hospital before the age of 25 years

   c. Men are more likely to experience impairment due to negative symptoms

   d. Its onset is earlier in men than in women

   e. Women show a bimodal distribution, with the second peak occurring in middle age (KS)

110. In which of the following populations is the prevalence of schizophrenia approximately 12%?

   a. Children of two parents with schizophrenia

   b. Dizygotic twins of parents with schizophrenia

   c. The general population

   d. Monozygotic twins of parents with schizophrenia

   e. Non-twin siblings of patients with schizophrenia (KS)

111. All of the following are excellent candidate genes for schizophrenia except:

   a. COMT

   b. DISC 1

   c. GRM 3

   d. 5-HTTLPR

   e. NRG 1 (KS)

112. Which of the following statements about the neuropathology of schizophrenia is true?

   a. Anterior cingulate basal ganglia thalamocortical circuit dysfunction underlies its negative symptom pathology

   b. It involves a decreased number of D_2 receptors in the caudate

   c. It involves an increase in the size of the parahippocampal gyrus

   d. The medial dorsal nucleus of the thalamus shows a reduced number of neurons

   e. It involves reduced symmetry of the frontotemporal but not the occipital lobes (KS)

113. All of the following statements about migration are true except:

   a. Excluding African-Caribbean people, in the UK the risk of bipolar disorder among migrants is reduced to insignificant levels

   b. The mean relative risk of any mood disorder among migrants does not depend on the relative risk among the African-Caribbean population

   c. The mean risk of developing bipolar disorder among migrants is 2.47

   d. The relative risk of developing schizophrenia in people with a family history of migration is 2.9

   e. White people with bipolar disorder present more often with hypomanic symptoms than do others (BJP 2007)

114. The presence of mood-incongruent psychotic features increases with evidence for linkage on which of the following chromosomes?

a. 1q21

b. 3q21

c. 9q21

d. 9p21

e. 13q21 (BJP 2007)

115. All of the following are statements about factors involved in inhibition and timing in cortical circuits except:

a. Interneuron alterations in schizophrenia are likely to have substantial effects on cognitive processes

b. The IPSPs generated by non-FS neurons reflect the perisomatic location of the synaptic contacts

c. Some interneurons contain somatostatin

d. Some interneurons express the calcium-binding protein calretinin

e. Synapses formed by PV neurons are found at or close to pyramidal cell bodies (BJP 2007)

116. All of the following statements about social problem-solving therapy for personality disorders are true except:

a. It aims to improve social competence

b. It can be offered as a brief intervention

c. It has been evaluated as a treatment for self-harm

d. Problem solving with psychoeducation reduces anger expression

e. It produces a significant improvement on measures of service use (BJP 2007)

117. All of the following statements about bibliotherapy in the treatment of social phobia are true except:

   a. The amount of reading is not related to outcomes of bibliotherapy

   b. Bibliotherapy is a successful treatment for anxiety disorders

   c. People with anxiety disorders prefer to deal with difficulties themselves

   d. Self-help shows sustained benefits in the treatment of social phobia

   e. Therapist-augmented bibliotherapy is effective for social phobia (BJP 2007)

118. All of the following statements about sleep in affective disorders are true except:

   a. Abnormal sleep patterns are associated with poor responses to psychotherapy

   b. Abnormal sleep patterns involve decreased phasic REM sleep

   c. Depression is associated with an increase in nocturnal arousal

   d. There is an increased core body temperature

   e. There is a reduction in the first period of non-REM sleep (KS)

119. Which of the following statements about brain imaging in affective disorders is true?

   a. It involves a decreased frequency of hyperintensities in the subcortical region in depression

   b. A decrease in glucose metabolism is associated with intrusive ruminations during depressive episodes

   c. It involves more greatly decreased metabolism in the right than in the left anterior brain in depression

   d. It involves increased caudate nuclear volume in depression

   e. The right prefrontal cortex is implicated in avoidance behaviours (KS)

120. The BCR gene is located on chromosome:

   a. 18p

   b. 21p

   c. 22p

   d. 21q

   e. 22q (KS)

121. Which of the following statements about dysthymic disorders is true?

   a. Dysthymia is common among 1–2% of the general population

   b. Dysthmic disorders involve increased REM latency

   c. A major defence mechanism is reaction formation

   d. Around 5–10% of those with childhood onset progress to manic or hypomanic episodes post-puberty

   e. Around 10% of those who have dysthmic disorders progress to bipolar type 1 disorder (KS)

122. An understanding of childhood disappointments as antecedents to adult depression can be gained through:

    a. Behaviour therapy

    b. Cognitive therapy

    c. Family therapy

    d. Interpersonal therapy

    e. Insight-oriented psychotherapy (KS)

123. All of the following statements about cyclothymic disorder are true except:

    a. Around 3–5% of all psychiatric outpatients have cyclothymia

    b. Around 25% of all patients with this disorder have an onset between the ages of 15 and 25 years

    c. The cyclothymic state is postulated to be the ego's attempt to overcome a punitive superego

    d. The female:male ratio for this disorder is 3:2

    e. Its lifetime prevalence is 1% (KS)

124. Which of the following statements about anxiety disorders is true?

    a. β-Carboline-3-carboxylic acid produces anxiety symptoms through activity on the GABA receptor

    b. CRH activates endocrine programmes for reproduction

    c. The NPY-Y2 receptor is implicated in the anxiogenic effects of neuropeptide Y

    d. Panic disorder is provoked by α_2-adrenoceptor agonists

    e. Stress reduces serotonin turnover in the amygdala (KS)

125. What is the term used for the requirement that the patient must tell everything that comes into their head?

   a. Analyst as mirror

   b. The fundamental rule

   c. The principle of evenly suspended attention

   d. The rule of abstinence

   e. Transference (KS)

126. The risk of OCD in the general population is:

   a. 0.1–0.5%

   b. 0.5–1.0%

   c. 1.0–1.5%

   d. 1.5–3%

   e. 3–5% (KS)

127. The most effective instruments in biofeedback include all of the following except:

   a. EEG

   b. EMG

   c. GSR

   d. Thermistor

   e. The Visual Analogue Scale (KS)

128. What is the term used for having patients direct their attention to specific bodily areas and hear themselves think certain phrases that reflect a relaxed state?

   a. Adaptation of progressive muscular relaxation

   b. Applied relaxation

   c. Applied tension

   d. Autogenic therapy

   e. Biofeedback (KS)

129. What is the term used for the step of applied relaxation in which patients relax just before entering the target situation, and stay in the situation for 10 to 15 minutes?

   a. Application training

   b. Cue-controlled relaxation

   c. Differential relaxation

   d. Progressive relaxation

   e. Release-only relaxation (KS)

130. What is the term used for the technique in which patients act out real-life problems under a therapist's observation or direction?

   a. Assertiveness training

   b. Behaviour rehearsal

   c. Psychodrama

   d. Social skills training

   e. Therapeutic graded exposure (KS)

Paper 5

1. Which of the following statements about the psychological treatment of premenstrual syndrome is true?
   a. Cognitive therapy is superior to information-focused therapy
   b. Combining fluoxetine and CBT is more effective than either treatment alone
   c. The National Association for Premenstrual Syndrome is run by patient-only groups
   d. Relaxation training is superior to coping-skills training
   e. Support groups have a good level of evidentiary support (APT 2007)

2. All of the following statements about suicide and antidepressants are true except:
   a. Anxiety disorder is a high-risk factor for suicidal acts for patients who are taking antidepressants
   b. The natural history of the disorder accounts for up to 10% of the placebo response
   c. The risk of suicidal acts for patients taking fluoxetine is 1.9 relative to those taking a placebo
   d. The CI for risk of suicidal acts for patients with bulimia who are taking fluoxetine is 0.3–6.9
   e. The risk of suicidal acts for patients taking SSRIs is 1.6 relative to those taking other antidepressants (APT 2006)

3. All of the following statements about the cognitive–behavioural therapy model for OCD are true except:

   a. According to this model, intrusive thoughts are universal, with a content indistinguishable from that of clinical obsessions

   b. Avoidance is not a part of the definition of OCD

   c. Excessive attentional bias on monitoring intrusive thoughts is specific to OCD

   d. Rumination covers both the obsession and any accompanying mental compulsion

   e. Thought–action fusion is also known as magical thinking (APT 2007)

4. Mrs Bentley is being considered for CBT for OCD. All of the following aspects are related to her treatment except:

   a. Combining actual and imagined exposure is superior to actual exposure alone

   b. The degree of family involvement is an area to be covered in the assessment

   c. In response prevention, patients are never forced to stop a compulsion

   d. The Obsessive-Compulsive Inventory is an objectively rated tool

   e. Prolonged exposure and response-prevention sessions with frequent homework will result in symptom reduction (APT 2007)

5. All of the following statements about the practice of psychological therapies for OCD are true except:

   a. Among those who are adherent to therapy, approximately 75% show improvement

   b. CBT is superior to exposure and response prevention

   c. Challenging a patient's appraisal of intrusive thoughts is associated with less success than challenging their content

   d. Hazardous CBT involves the therapist becoming engaged in subtle requests for reassurance

   e. Around 25% of all patients refuse or drop out from exposure and response prevention (APT 2007)

6. Mrs Schmidt is being considered for CBT for OCD. The psychologist in your team wants to know from your assessment the factors for her prognosis. The poor prognostic factors include all of the following except:

   a. Comorbid schizoid personality

   b. Expressed hostility from family members

   c. Hoarding

   d. Overvalued ideation

   e. Severe avoidance (APT 2007)

7. All of the following statements about CBT for paranoia are true except:

   a. Clinicians need to be flexible with regard to the length of the sessions

   b. The evidence is strongest for negative symptoms such as apathy

   c. It is an exploratory approach

   d. It reduces recovery time for acute psychosis

   e. Self-help includes testing out suspicious thoughts (APT 2006)

8. Which of the following is an ineffective remedy in the treatment of anxiety?

a. *Crataegus oxyacantha*

b. *Melissa officinalis*

c. *Passiflora incarnate*

d. *Piper methysticum*

e. *Valeriana officinalis* (APT 2007)

9. The herbal remedy that interacts with phenothiazide to cause epileptic seizures is:

a. Evening primrose oil

b. Kava

c. Lemon balm

d. St John's Wort

e. Valerian (APT 2007)

10. The herbal remedy that interacts with levodopa to produce extrapyramidal symptoms is:

a. Evening primrose oil

b. Kava

c. Maidenhair tree

d. St John's Wort

e. Valerian (APT 2007)

11. Which of the following is the symptom with the highest frequency among core manic symptoms in hypomania?

a. Decreased sleep

b. Disinhibition

c. Increased activity

d. Increased plans or ideas

e. Increased talkativeness (APT 2006)

12. All of the following are substances associated with hypomania except:

    a. Amphetamine

    b. Alcohol

    c. Cannabis

    d. Cocaine

    e. MDMA (APT 2006)

13. All of the following correlations are true except:

    a. Chronic fatigue syndrome – reduced activity in orbitofrontal cortex

    b. Chronic functional pain – down-regulation of anterior cingulate cortex

    c. Eating disorder – activation of the right amygdala

    d. Functional angina – activation of anterior cingulate cortex

    e. Somatisation – reduced metabolism in bilateral caudate nuclei (APT 2006)

14. All of the following associations between stroke and mood disorder are true except:

    a. Antidepressants are effective in treating emotionalism irrespective of a diagnosis of depression

    b. Bromocriptine aggravates apathy following a stroke

    c. The standardised mortality rate from suicide following a stroke increases by threefold

    d. There is more evidence of lability of mood in mood disorders associated with a stroke

    e. Tricyclic antidepressants are more effective than SSRIs (APT 2006)

15. Which of the following statements about epilepsy is true?

    a. CBT is ineffective in the treatment of non-epileptic seizures

    b. Episodic psychosis is unrelated to prescribed drug use

    c. The lifetime prevalence of panic disorder is 10%

    d. The prevalence of neuropsychiatric disorder in people with epilepsy is 3%

    e. Up to 50% of people who are referred to specialist epilepsy centres have non-epileptic episodes (APT 2006)

16. Which of the following statements about neuropsychiatric disorders and Parkinson's disease is true?

    a. Anxiety is common in older patients with Parkinson's disease

    b. Depression is common among women patients

    c. Delusions are found in 1% of patients with Parkinson's disease

    d. The prevalence of all psychiatric syndromes among patients with Parkinson's disease is 30%

    e. Around 5% of patients with Parkinson's disease with no dementia have cognitive impairment (APT 2006)

17. All of the following statements about drug treatment and Parkinson's disease are correct except:

    a. Clozapine at a dose greater than 100 mg/day is the treatment of choice for psychosis

    b. Dopamine agonist treatment is associated with hypomania in pre-existing bipolar affective disorder

    c. Dopaminergic drugs are associated with psychosis

    d. SSRIs exacerbate extrapyramidal symptoms

    e. Tricyclic antidepressants may improve motor symptoms (APT 2006)

18. Which of the following statements about smoking cessation treatments is correct?

    a. Bupropion induces weight gain

    b. The gold standard is pharmacotherapy plus individual or group support

    c. Pre-loading with nicotine replacement therapy reduces cessation rates

    d. Nortriptyline is less effective than SSRIs

    e. Varenicline is less effective than bupropion (APT 2008)

19. Which of the following statements about nicotine replacement therapy (NRT) is correct?

    a. Its nasal spray form is not available in the UK

    b. The risk ratio of abstinence for any form of NRT relative to control is 1.58

    c. The risk ratio is significantly greater for gum than for lozenges

    d. A single form of replacement is more effective than combined forms

    e. Using NRT for short periods before quitting delays abstinence (APT 2008)

20. Which of the following statements about pharmacological treatments for smoking is true?

    a. Carbamazepine decreases the level of hydroxybupropion

    b. Nortriptyline's mode of action is independent of its antidepressant effect

    c. Rimonabant is a selective μ-receptor agonist

    d. The most common side-effect of bupropion is sleepiness

    e. Varenicline is a nicotinic receptor antagonist (APT 2008)

21. All of the following statements about psychological treatments for smoking are true except:

    a. The evidence of success of brief interventions provided by nurses is weak

    b. Exercise has a positive effect on cigarette cravings

    c. Group therapy is more effective than self-help

    d. Self-help material has an additive effect when used alongside NRT

    e. Simple advice from a physician has a significant odds ratio of 1.74 (APT 2008)

22. Which of the following statements about smoking and mental illnesses is true?

    a. The daily consumption of 15 or more cigarettes per day is required for the metabolism of mirtazapine

    b. During smoking cessation, doses of clozapine but not of olanzapine need to be reduced to 75% to prevent toxicity

    c. The incremental cost per life-year saved for NRT is £500

    d. The use of both NRT and CBT doubles the cessation rates for patients with depression

    e. Although bupropion reduces relapse rates, it is associated with the worsening of psychotic symptoms (APT 2008)

23. Which of the following statements about alcohol and EEG is true?

    a. Chronic alcoholism shows similar changes to intoxication

    b. Intoxication is associated with fast activity in the temporal area

    c. Intoxication is associated with decreased beta waves

    d. It takes 6 to 12 months for slow-wave sleep to become normal following abstinence

    e. Withdrawal is associated with slow waves (SBN)

24. Which of the following statements about the NICE guidelines for OCD is correct?

   a. Adults who show mild impairment but are unable to engage in low, intense CBT should not be considered for high, intense CBT

   b. Adults with moderate functional impairment should be offered CBT combined with SSRI treatment

   c. Adding an SSRI to CBT is contraindicated for children aged between 8 and 11 years

   d. Initial offers of treatment should include exposure and response prevention

   e. Step 5 involves inpatient treatment (www.nice.org.uk)

25. According to the NICE guidelines for OCD, all of the following statements are true except:

   a. Therapists need to advise patients that there is no convincing evidence for the effectiveness of psychoanalysis

   b. Therapists need to consider giving cognitive therapy in addition to exposure and response prevention, to enhance long-term symptom reduction

   c. Therapists need to consider cognitive therapy for patients who refuse to engage in exposure and response prevention

   d. Therapists need to consider using rewards for motivation

   e. Therapists need to discourage patients' families from using exposure and response prevention should new symptoms emerge (www.nice.org.uk)

26. According to the NICE guidelines, which of the following statements is true?

    a. Therapists need to carry out an ECG before commencing clomipramine

    b. Therapists need to inform patients that it might take up to 12 weeks for an improvement to be noticed

    c. Drug treatment may be continued for up to 12 months if it is effective

    d. SSRI treatment for children should be continued for 6 months after remission if a response is observed

    e. Therapists should offer clomipramine as a first-line drug treatment for adults (www.nice.org.uk)

27. All of the following statements about the NICE guidelines for bipolar affective disorder are true except:

    a. If a patient is taking an antidepressant at the onset of manic symptoms, that antidepressant should not be stopped abruptly

    b. If antipsychotics are ineffective in the treatment of mania, augmenting them with valproate should be considered

    c. The guidelines recommend olanzapine for long-term treatment

    d. Patients should not routinely continue antidepressants as a long-term treatment

    e. Risperidone is licensed for the acute treatment of mania (www.nice.org.uk)

28. Which of the following does the angular gyrus receive?

    a. Auditory input

    b. Smell input

    c. Somaesthetic input

    d. Taste input

    e. Visual input (TN)

29. All of the following are parts of the limbic lobe except the:
    a. Cingulate gyrus
    b. Parahippocampal gyrus
    c. Paraolfactory gyrus
    d. Precuneus
    e. Preterminal gyrus (TN)

30. Afferent fibres from the thalamus are found in the:
    a. External granular layer
    b. External pyramidal layer
    c. Fusiform layer
    d. Internal pyramidal layer
    e. Molecular layer (TN)

31. Stellate neurons are found in the:
    a. External granular layer
    b. External pyramidal layer
    c. Fusiform layer
    d. Internal pyramidal layer
    e. Molecular layer (TN)

32. The right and left amygdalas are connected by the:
    a. Anterior commissure
    b. Genu of corpus callosum
    c. Hippocampal commissure
    d. Posterior commissure
    e. Rostrum of the corpus callosum (TN)

33. Mr Bainbridge presents with right hemiparesis, loss of proprioception and loss of his vibratory sense. To which of the following is this due?

    a. The left anterior spinal artery at the medulla

    b. The left anterior spinal artery at the spinal level

    c. A left posterior spinal-artery occlusion

    d. The right anterior spinal artery at the spinal level

    e. A right posterior spinal-artery occlusion (TN)

34. Which of the following is predominantly released by the pyramidal cells in the cortex?

    a. Acetylcholine

    b. Dopamine

    c. Glutamate

    d. Glycine

    e. Serotonin (TN)

35. Which of the following is the function of the red nucleus?

    a. Coordination of eye and neck movements

    b. Orientation of the head

    c. The reflex movements of the axial and limb musculature

    d. Sensory modulation

    e. The voluntary movements of the upper limb muscles (TN)

36. In which of the following are the pyramidal cells that contribute to the corticospinal and corticobulbar tracts situated?

    a. Layer I

    b. Layer II

    c. Layer III

    d. Layer IV

    e. Layer V (TN)

37. All of the following statements about the premotor cortex are true except:

   a. Its key function is in the planning phase of motor activity

   b. It involves area 6

   c. It is on the lateral aspect of the frontal lobe

   d. Once an intended activity begins, its activity continues to increase

   e. Its principal function is the control of axial and proximal limb musculature (TN)

38. Mr Bainbridge presents with a wrinkled forehead, raised eyebrow, drooping eyelid, dilated pupil, and downward and abducted eye on the left half of his face. Which of the following does the lesion involve?

   a. The left abducens nerve

   b. The left oculomotor nerve

   c. The left trochlear nerve

   d. The right facial nerve

   e. The right oculomotor nerve (TN)

39. Mr Bainbridge presents with a diplopia that becomes very prominent when descending stairs and while reading. It also tilts his head to the right side. This could be due to a lesion involving:

   a. The left trochlear nerve

   b. The left trochlear nucleus

   c. The right abducens nerve

   d. The right facial nerve

   e. The right trochlear nerve (TN)

40. Which of the following is mediated by the mesencephalic nucleus of the trigeminal nerve?

    a. The contraction of the muscles of mastication

    b. The jaw-jerk reflex

    c. Pain and thermal sensation from the mandibular division of the nerve

    d. Taste from the anterior two-thirds of the tongue

    e. Touch and pressure sensation from the maxillary division of the nerve (TN)

41. On eye testing, Mr Bainbridge can gaze to the right with no apparent difficulty. On attempting to gaze to the left, his right eye cannot move inward and his left eye moves outward. He is able to look at a pen placed directly in front of him with no difficulty. The lesion involves the:

    a. Right abducens

    b. Right medial longitudinal fasciculus

    c. Right ophthalmic nerve

    d. Right optic nerve

    e. Right trochlear nerve (TN)

42. All of the following statements about the taste pathway are true except:

    a. The anterior two-thirds of the tongue are supplied by the facial nerve

    b. The fibres from the ventroposteromedial nucleus end in the parietal operculum

    c. The nodose ganglion receives the fibres from the posterior third of the tongue

    d. Some fibres from the solitary nucleus pass to the parabrachial nucleus

    e. Taste fibres pass through the posterior limb of the internal capsule (TN)

43. Which of the following statements about the cytoarchitecture of the cerebral cortex is true?

a. Aspiny cells release glutamate

b. The cells of Martinotti are bipolar

c. Fusiform cells have their dendritic projections to deep cortical layers

d. The horizontal cells of Cajal are situated in deep cortical layers

e. Pyramidal cells release aspartate (TN)

44. All of the following statements about the cell layers of the neo-cortex are true except:

a. The external granular layer consists mainly of stellate cells

b. The internal pyramidal layer is the source of the majority of the corticofugal fibres

c. Layer IV is the main efferent station of the cerebral cortex

d. The pyramidal cell axons of the external pyramidal layer are the principal source of the corticocortical fibres

e. The most numerous cells in the plexiform layer are the horizontal cells of Cajal (TN)

45. The arcuate fasciculus is part of the:

a. Inferior longitudinal fibres

b. Inferior occipitofrontal fasciculus

c. Short-association fibres

d. Superior occipitofrontal fasciculus

e. Superior longitudinal fasciculus (TN)

46. All of the following statements about the internal capsule are true except:

    a. Its anterior limb includes corticothalamic radiations

    b. Its genu transmits corticobulbar fibres

    c. It has sub- and retrolenticular limbs

    d. Its posterior limb is between the head of the caudate nucleus and the lentiform nucleus

    e. Its retrolenticular limb carries visual information (TN)

47. All of the following statements about the motor cortex are true except:

    a. Part of the precentral gyrus controlling the movements of the tongue is located at its inferior aspect

    b. The premotor cortex receives fibres from the cerebellum through the ventral lateral nucleus of the thalamus

    c. Its primary motor area corresponds to Brodmann's area 4

    d. Its secondary motor cortex is localised exclusively to the frontal lobe

    e. Its supplementary motor area receives input from the basal ganglia (TN)

48. Which of the following equations regarding the composition of intracellular fluid is accurate?

    a. $Na^+ = 152$ mmol/L

    b. $Cl^- = 117$ mmol/L

    c. $HCO_3^- = 27$ mmol/L

    d. Proteins = 74 mmol/L

    e. $Ca^{2+} = 5$ mmol/L (SBN)

49. All of the following statements about cell membranes are true except:

    a. They behave as if there were pores

    b. They are permeable to large molecules

    c. They are permeable to lipophilic substances

    d. They are permeable to water

    e. They are selectively permeable to ions (SBN)

50. Which of the following statements about action potentials is true?

    a. At equilibrium, the electrical force that prevents an efflux of potassium ions is opposed by the concentration gradient that promotes efflux

    b. There are two different types of calcium channels

    c. $E_{Cl} = -95\,mV$

    d. Their refractory period is due to the voltage-dependent inactivation of the K^+ channels

    e. A sodium pump contributes $-127\,mV$ to their resting membrane potential (SBN)

51. The fibres with the fastest conduction velocity are the:

    a. Aα fibres

    b. Aβ fibres

    c. Aγ fibres

    d. Aδ fibres

    e. C fibres (SBN)

52. Which of the following statements about higher-order somato-sensory processing is true?

    a. Its large peripheral innervations have a small cortical representation

    b. Its lateral inhibition involves GABA-mediated inhibition by interneurons on adjacent second-order neurons

    c. Its lateral inhibition is a mechanism for limiting the spread of excitation between couples inputs

    d. Its lateral inhibition is one form of feedback inhibition

    e. There are only two different representations of the body's surface in the cortex (SBN)

53. All of the following are features of surface dyslexia except:

    a. A breakdown of whole-word reading

    b. Difficulty in reading irregularly spelt words

    c. An inability to read non-words

    d. A lesion in the left temporoparietal region

    e. Making phonologically possible errors

54. Which of the following is a characteristic feature of peripheral dysgraphia?

    a. Better concrete than abstract spelling

    b. A breakdown of the lexical route for spelling

    c. Oral spelling remaining intact with defective copying

    d. Semantic errors

    e. Being unable to spell non-words (CA)

55. All of the following lesions are correctly matched except:

a. Acalculia – left angular gyrus

b. Alexia without agraphia – left medial occipital lobe

c. Dyspraxic dysgraphia – dominant temporal lobe

d. Lexical dysgraphia – left temporoparietal region

e. Neglect dysphasia – right hemisphere lesion (CA)

56. All of the following tests are correctly matched except:

a. The ability to point to numbers test – dyscalculia

b. The Cambridge Semantic Battery – visual agnosias

c. The meaningful and meaningless gesture test – sensory neglect

d. The single-letter identification test – dyslexia

e. The spontaneous writing of sentences test – dysgraphia (CA)

57. Mr Bainbridge presents with a breakdown of fine motor coordination. He has difficulty copying meaningless hand gestures, but can copy meaningful ones. This is:

a. Conceptual apraxia

b. Ideational apraxia

c. Ideomotor apraxia

d. Limb kinetic apraxia

e. Oral apraxia (CA)

58. Which of the following statements about spasmodic torticollis is true?

a. Its annual incidence is 1 in 1 000 000

b. Anticholinergic treatment is effective in more than 50% of patients with this condition

c. Botulinum toxin is a rare cause of spasmodic torticollis

d. It is the most common focal dystonia

e. Remission occurs in 40% of patients with this condition (SBN)

59. Which of the following statements about neuroleptic-induced movement disorders is true?

a. α but not β adrenoceptor antagonists are useful in the treatment of akathisia

b. Dopamine agonists worsen the symptoms of neuroleptic malignant syndrome

c. The incidence of acute dystonia can be as high as 10% for high-potency neuroleptics

d. Fewer than 50% of those affected with tardive dyskinesia have symptoms restricted to their face

e. Tremors are the first feature to develop in drug-induced parkinsonism (SBN)

60. Mr Bainbridge presents with daytime somnolence associated with hypoxia and recurrent waking during the night. The diagnosis is:

a. Alzheimer's dementia

b. Cataplexy

c. Kleine–Levin syndrome

d. Narcolepsy

e. Pickwickian syndrome (SBN)

61. Mr Bainbridge presents with narcolepsy, sleep paralysis and hypnogogic hallucinations. This is:

   a. Ganser syndrome

   b. Gelineau syndrome

   c. Kleine–Levin syndrome

   d. Kluver–Bucy syndrome

   e. None of the above (SBN)

62. All of the following are disorders of neural-tube defects except:

   a. Chiari malformation

   b. Encephalocele

   c. Holoprosencephaly

   d. Meningocele

   e. Spina bifida (SBN)

63. Which of the following conditions results from a persistent infection by the measles virus with inclusions in neurons and oligodendrocytes?

   a. Binswanger's disease

   b. Lacunar disease

   c. Subacute sclerosing panencephalitis

   d. Perivenous encephalomyelitis

   e. Progressive multifocal leukoencephalopathy (SBN)

64. All of the following statements about neurosyphilis are true except:

    a. There is dorsal column involvement that leads to loss of proprioception

    b. Optic atrophy may occur

    c. The pupils are small

    d. The pupils respond to light but not accommodation

    e. Its vascular forms may be associated with raised intracranial pressure (SBN)

65. All of the following statements about neurofibrillary tangles are true except:

    a. They are absent in progressive supranuclear palsy

    b. They can be found in the locus coeruleus

    c. They consist of intracellular paired helical filaments

    d. They are formed by abnormal phosphorylation of the tau protein

    e. They are present in post-encephalitic parkinsonism (SBN)

66. Swollen cortical pyramidal cells are seen in:

    a. Alzheimer's disease

    b. Creutzfeldt–Jacob disease

    c. Huntington's disease

    d. Parkinson's disease

    e. Pick's disease (SBN)

67. In which of the following is the 'fried-egg' appearance seen?

    a. Anaplastic astrocytomas

    b. Astrocytomas

    c. Ependymomas

    d. Glioblastoma multiforme

    e. Oligodendrogliomas (SBN)

68. The expression of steroid receptors in tumours can be studied using:

    a. Indomethacin

    b. Reboxetine

    c. Riluzole

    d. Tamoxifen

    e. Viloxazine (SBN)

69. Which of the following is the enzyme that inactivates circulating cortisol in tissues that express mineralocorticoid receptors?

    a. 9-hydroxysteroid dehydrogenase

    b. 9-cortisol cyclase

    c. 11-hydroxysteroid dehydrogenase

    d. 11-cortisol cyclase

    e. 11-hydroxysteroid decarboxylase (SBN)

70. All of the following are associated with insulin resistance except:

    a. Acanthosis nigricans

    b. Hypertriglyceridaemia

    c. Lipodystrophy

    d. Polycystic ovaries

    e. Testicular feminisation (SBN)

71. All of the following statements about insulin-like growth factor (IGF) binding proteins are true except:

    a. IGF-1 has a 60% homology with proinsulin

    b. IGF-1 mediates the functions of growth hormone

    c. IGF binding protein 1 (IGFBP-1) binds to both IGF-1 and IGF-2

    d. IGFBP-1 shows diurnal variation

    e. IGFBP-1 shows a gradual decline from childhood to puberty (SBN)

72. Which of the following controls the posterior pituitary?

    a. The ventroposterolateral nucleus

    b. The magnocellular paraventricular nucleus

    c. The preoptic nucleus

    d. The suprachiasmatic nucleus

    e. All of the above (SBN)

73. All of the following statements about fragile X syndrome are true except:

    a. It is associated with a loss of expression of the FMR2 gene

    b. It is associated with attentional difficulties and hyperactivity

    c. It is the single commonest known inherited cause of mental retardation

    d. Its mutation involves CGG repeats within the first exon of the FMR1 gene

    e. The rate of fragile X syndrome is higher among children with autism than among those with a learning disability (PG)

74. As which of the following does the microdeletion of chromosome 7q11 present?

   a. Angelman syndrome

   b. Di George syndrome

   c. Smith–Magenis syndrome

   d. Turner's syndrome

   e. Williams syndrome (PG)

75. Which of the syndromes listed below is characterised by a prevalence of 1 to 2 per 2000, males affected by it being characteristically tall and having lower IQs than the general population, and an association with minor criminality?

   a. Klinefelter's syndrome

   b. Prader–Willi syndrome

   c. Smith–Magenis syndrome

   d. Turner's syndrome

   e. XYY syndrome (PG)

76. Bainbridge Junior presents with a mild learning difficulty, a cleft palate, hypocalcaemia, and speech and swallowing difficulties. This is a presentation of:

   a. Angelman syndrome

   b. Di George syndrome

   c. Smith–Magenis syndrome

   d. Turner's syndrome

   e. Williams syndrome (PG)

77. Bainbridge Junior presents with onychotillomania, polyembolokoilamania and self-hugging. This is a presentation of:

  a. Angelman syndrome

  b. Di George syndrome

  c. Smith–Magenis syndrome

  d. Turner's syndrome

  e. Williams syndrome (PG)

78. Which of the following statements about excitatory amino acids is true?

  a. Around 20% of all synapses use glutamate as a transmitter

  b. Glutaminase converts glutamate to glutamine

  c. The hippocampal pyramidal cells use glutamate as a transmitter

  d. Glutamate is converted to glutamine in neurons

  e. In rough endoplasmic reticulum, glutamate is formed from glutamine (N)

79. All of the following statements about inhibitory amino acids are true except:

  a. Cerebellar Purkinje cells use GABA as a neurotransmitter

  b. GABA is synthesised from glutamate by glutamic acid decarboxylase

  c. The glycine receptor is activated by strychnine

  d. The Renshaw cells of the spinal cord use glycine as a neurotransmitter

  e. Vigabatrin inhibits the catabolism of GABA to succinic semialdehyde (N)

80. All of the following statements about dopamine are true except:

    a. Around 80% of all dopaminergic neurons are found in the substantia nigra

    b. Aldehyde dehydrogenase metabolises dopamine to homovanillic acid

    c. The amacrine cells of the retina use dopamine as a neurotransmitter

    d. Dopaminergic neurons are unmyelinated

    e. The hydroxylation of tyrosine is the rate-limiting step in the synthesis of dopamine (N)

81. Which of the following statements about dopamine is true?

    a. D_1 receptors are autoreceptors

    b. The D_2 family is coupled to G_s

    c. D_3 receptors are postsynaptic autoreceptors

    d. Striatum expresses D_4 receptors

    e. The vesicular monoamine transporter is blocked by reserpine (N)

82. Which of the following statements about noradrenaline is true?

    a. Amphetamine increases stores of noradrenaline

    b. DOPEG excretion is used as a measure of noradrenaline turnover

    c. The noradrenaline transporter is a non-saturable Na^+/Cl^--dependent transporter

    d. The locus coeruleus contributes to the dorsal noradrenergic bundle

    e. Phenylethanolamine N-methyl transferase is the rate-limiting factor in the synthesis of norepinephrine (N)

83. The process that involves two different chromosomes fusing at or near the centromere is called:

    a. Deletion

    b. Duplication

    c. Inversion

    d. Robertsonian translocation

    e. Substitution (PG)

84. The mechanism by which the variation in the rate at which a gene is expressed can be inherited in the absence of a change in the primary DNA sequence is called:

    a. Anticipation

    b. Epigenetic inheritance

    c. A frame-shift mutation

    d. A trinucleotide repeat

    e. Uniparental isodisomy (PG)

85. In which of the following is methylation involved?

    a. Angelman syndrome

    b. Rett syndrome

    c. Smith–Magenis syndrome

    d. Turner's syndrome

    e. Williams syndrome (PG)

86. In which of the following is anticipation seen?

    a. Angelman syndrome

    b. Fragile X syndrome

    c. Smith–Magenis syndrome

    d. Turner's syndrome

    e. Williams syndrome (PG)

87. In which of the following is uniparental isodisomy involving maternal chromosome 15 seen?

    a. Angelman syndrome

    b. Prader–Willi syndrome

    c. Smith–Magenis syndrome

    d. Turner's syndrome

    e. Williams syndrome (PG)

88. Which of the following statements about brain-derived neuro-trophic factor (BDNF) and bipolar disorder is true?

    a. The BDNF gene is associated with the early onset of bipolar disorder

    b. GT(n) polymorphism is not associated with rapid cycling disorder

    c. Mania may be caused by under-activity of the central BDNF function

    d. Val66Met polymorphism is associated with susceptibility to bipolar disorder

    e. Val66Met polymorphism is associated with susceptibility to rapid cycling (BJP 2006)

89. All of the following statements about borderline personality disorder (BPD) are true except:

    a. Around 75% of people with BPD show remission within 6 years after presentation

    b. Individuals with BPD have a hyperactive attachment system

    c. Psychiatrists must take an expert role rather than an inquisitive stance in treating BPD

    d. The recurrence rate of BPD is no more than 10% over 6 years

    e. BPD patients' relative risk of attempted suicide following treatment with dialectical behaviour therapy is –1.38 (BJP 2006)

90. All of the following statements about brain volume in first-episode schizophrenia are true except:

    a. The average volume deficit is less than 3%

    b. The left ventricle is more enlarged than the right ventricle

    c. No significant long-term change has been observed in the volumetric deficits seen at diagnosis involving the insula and the thalamus

    d. It involves a reduction in whole brain volume but not in the volume of the hippocampus

    e. Ventricular volume is increased (BJP 2006)

91. Which of the following statements about coronary heart disease and severe mental illness (SMI) is true?

    a. Coronary heart disease is second only to suicide when the mortality rates from different causes are compared

    b. Excess coronary heart disease is completely accounted for by a combination of medication and socio-economic circumstances

    c. The mortality rate from coronary heart disease has decreased with the advent of atypical antipsychotics

    d. The odds ratio of the association between SMI and HDL-cholesterol is 4.0

    e. There is no significant association between SMI and diabetes (BJP 2006)

92. All of the following statements about CBT are true except:

a. Adjunctive CBT is only of benefit to people who have had fewer than 12 episodes of bipolar affective disorder

b. A long-term study of the use of CBT for treating comorbid schizophrenia and substance misuse found that it had no effect on the percentage of days of abstinence

c. CBT can reduce interpersonal difficulty among people at high risk for psychosis

d. CBT is effective for problems associated with amphetamine use

e. A reduction in compliance with command hallucination with a reduction in voice activity occurs following CBT for psychosis (BJP 2006)

93. Which of the following statements about the epidemiology of common mental illnesses is true?

a. In the UK, household income and geographical localisation have a significant effect on people's mental health

b. Quantifying between-place differences using population density alone is the best way of interpreting the role of geographical localisation in mental health

c. Socioeconomic factors have a greater impact on the duration of episodes of mental illness than the time of their onset

d. Suicide rates are higher in the urban areas of England but not of Wales

e. Those living in rural areas have better mental health than those living in non-rural areas (BJP 2006)

94. All of the following epidemiological observations are true except:

    a. Agoraphobia occurs at 2 per 100 person-years at risk

    b. Baseline agoraphobia without spontaneous panic disorder does not predict the first incidence of panic disorder

    c. Cluster B disorders are associated with early institutional care

    d. Other phobias predict the incidence of agoraphobia

    e. The prevalence of personality disorder is highest among men (BJP 2006)

95. Which of the following statements about the psychological impact of stillbirth is true?

    a. The father's psychological morbidity is not associated with the presence of other children in the family

    b. Stillbirth is a category C event for the development of PTSD in women

    c. Stillbirth is a risk factor for anxiety but not for depression among women during subsequent pregnancies

    d. Stillbirth is associated with prescribed drug use but not with alcohol use among fathers

    e. It involves a significant difference in trait anxiety between mothers and fathers, both antenatally and at follow-up (BJP 2006)

96. Which of the following statements about changes in grey matter is true?

    a. A dominant unilateral increase in the volume of putamen takes place in adolescents with Tourette's syndrome

    b. The dorsal striatum is impaired in the cortico–striatal–thalamic–cortical circuitry implicated in Tourette's syndrome

    c. Grey matter increases in the left hippocampus of adolescents with Tourette's syndrome

    d. A number of soft neurological signs are associated with a reduction in grey matter in the prefrontal cortex

    e. A number of soft neurological signs are associated with a reduction in grey matter in the lingual gyrus (BJP 2006)

97. All of the following statements about group therapies are true except:

    a. Group CBT has a significant impact on schizophrenia relapse rates

    b. Group CBT reduces feelings of hopelessness in patients with schizophrenia

    c. Group CBT reduces low self-esteem among patients with schizophrenia

    d. Group IPT has a significant effect on depression, which is maintained at 6-month follow-up

    e. Group psychoeducational interventions offered to women in primary care reduce depressive symptoms (BJP 2006)

98. All of the following statements about a synapse are true except:

a. Changes in the structure of synapses are mediated by growth factors

b. Conjoint synapses have both electrical and chemical characteristics

c. Nitric oxide, but not carbon monoxide, acts as a neurotransmitter in a synapse

d. The propagation of an action potential along an axon is an all-or-nothing phenomenon

e. The synaptic compartment represents less than 1% of the brain (KS)

99. Which of the following types of receptor is involved in seizures?

a. α_1

b. D_1

c. H_1

d. M_1

e. 5-HT_{1A} (KS)

100. Which of the following is the neurotransmitter in most primary afferent sensory neurons?

a. Acetylcholine

b. Corticotropin-releasing factor

c. Neuropeptide Y

d. Neurotensin

e. Substance P (KS)

101. All of the following statements about structural neuroimaging techniques are true except:

   a. Areas of the brain with an abnormally high water content appear brighter on a T2 image

   b. Bony structures absorb the largest amount of radiation during a CT scan

   c. CSF is dark on a T1 image

   d. FLAIR is useful for detecting sclerosis of the hippocampus caused by temporal lobe epilepsy

   e. MRI images are obtained in the axial and coronal planes but not in the sagittal plane (KS)

102. Which of the following statements about magnetic resonance spectroscopy (MRS) is true?

   a. Dopamine cannot be detected using MRS

   b. Just like MRI, MRS detects hydrogen nuclei only

   c. An MRS of hydrogen-1 nuclei is used to detect the pH of the different regions of the brain

   d. An MRS of hydrogen-1 nuclei is used to measure ATP

   e. The resolution of MRS is equal to that of PET (KS)

103. EEGs show increased alpha activity with the use of which of the following?

   a. Alcohol

   b. Barbiturates

   c. Caffeine

   d. Opioids

   e. Nicotine (KS)

104. An EEG pattern of increased alpha activity in the frontal area, but with overall slow alpha activity, is seen with the use of which of the following?

a. Alcohol

b. Barbiturates

c. Cocaine

d. Opioids

e. Nicotine (KS)

105. Which of the following is an EEG feature of cerebrovascular accidents?

a. A diffuse asynchronous high-voltage slowing

b. A diffuse generalised slowing of wake frequencies

c. Focal delta activity

d. Focal delta slowing

e. Triphasic waves (KS)

106. Which of the following is a steroid-like hormone?

a. ACTH

b. β-Endorphin

c. FSH

d. LH

e. Thyroxine (KS)

107. Which of the following is a research area that uses a range of bioinformatic approaches to analyse the expression and function of proteins within specific systems, cells or organisms?

    a. Epigenetics

    b. Linkage analysis

    c. Multifactorial analysis

    d. Polygenics

    e. Proteomics (KS)

108. Which of the following statements about the neuropathology of schizophrenia is true?

    a. A blunted prolactin response is seen in association with positive symptoms

    b. The brains of people with schizophrenia show lower levels of phosphomonoester compared with the general population

    c. People with schizophrenia have higher concentrations of n-acetyl aspartate in the hippocampus compared with the general population

    d. The neuropathology of schizophrenia involves increased levels of T-cell interleukin-2 production

    e. Around 25% of people with schizophrenia present with eye-movement dysfunction (KS)

109. All of the following factors are associated with a good prognosis in schizophrenia except:

    a. Symptoms of depressive disorder

    b. A family history of mood disorders

    c. A history of assaultiveness

    d. Being married

    e. Having positive symptoms (KS)

110. Which of the following statements about the comorbidities associated with schizophrenia is true?

    a. People with schizophrenia tend to have higher rates of chronic obstructive pulmonary disease than people in the general population, independent of smoking

    b. An inverse relationship exists between rheumatoid arthritis and schizophrenia

    c. A lack of awareness of a movement disorder is associated with a lack of insight into a primary psychiatric disorder

    d. Patients with schizophrenia are at no higher risk of HIV than the general population

    e. All of the above are true (KS)

111. All of the following are risk factors for suicide among inpatients with common mental illnesses except:

    a. Involvement with the police

    b. Previous suicidal behaviour

    c. The presence of hallucinations

    d. Suffering a recent bereavement

    e. Engaging in violence against property (BJP 2006)

112. All of the following are risk factors for suicide among patients discharged from hospital care except:

    a. A lack of continuity of care

    b. The lack of a social network

    c. Suicidal ideation prior to discharge

    d. Unemployment

    e. An unplanned discharge (BJP 2006)

113. Which of the following statements about schizoaffective disorder is true?

   a. The depressive type may be more common in young adults

   b. The lifetime prevalence of schizoaffective disorder is less than 0.5%

   c. Lithium is ineffective in the treatment of schizoaffective disorder

   d. Mood disorder dominance is associated with a poor prognosis

   e. The disorder's prevalence is significantly lower in married men than in women (KS)

114. Which of the following statements about delusional disorder is true?

   a. Its annual incidence is less than 1 case per 100 000 patients

   b. Its diagnostic criteria include the presence of a non-bizarre delusion for at least 3 months

   c. The mean age of onset is around 40 years

   d. More than 25% of its cases are reclassified as schizophrenia or a mood disorder at follow-up

   e. A slight male preponderance exists (KS)

115. All of the following statements about the aetiology of delusional disorder are true except:

   a. According to classic psychodynamic theory, the dynamics underlying the formation of delusions are independent of gender

   b. Family history is not significantly associated with delusional disorder

   c. The neurological conditions most commonly associated with delusional disorder involve the basal ganglia

   d. Reaction formation is a primary defence mechanism used by patients with delusional disorder

   e. Sensory isolation is associated with delusional disorder (KS)

116. Mr Bainbridge presents with a belief that his wife can assume the guise of strangers. This is called:

a. Capgras syndrome

b. Delusional intermetamorphosis

c. Folie impose

d. Fregoli's phenomenon

e. Illusion de sosies (KS)

117. All of the following personality disorders involve high susceptibility to developing psychotic symptoms except:

a. Borderline personality disorder

b. Antisocial personality disorder

c. Paranoid personality disorder

d. Schizoid personality disorder

e. Schizotypal personality disorder (KS)

118. All of the following statements about genetic factors in affective disorder are true except:

a. The monozygotic concordance rate for mood disorders is 70–90%

b. The presence of more severe illnesses in a family conveys a greater risk than other factors

c. The risk of a child having an affective disorder if one parent is affected is 10–25%

d. Twin-study findings show that genes account for only 30% of the aetiology of mood disorders

e. Unipolar disorder is the most common form of disorder in families of bipolar probands (KS)

119. The CREB1 locus is located on chromosome:

a. 1

b. 2

c. 18

d. 21

e. 22 (KS)

120. Which of the following statements about psychosocial factors in affective disorders is true?

a. The development of depression is associated with losing a parent before the age of 14 years

b. The environmental stressor that is most strongly associated with the prevention of remission is the loss of a partner

c. People who are unemployed are three times more likely to report symptoms of an episode of major depression than employed people

d. People with antisocial personality disorder are more predisposed to depression than people with anankastic personality disorder

e. People with a histrionic personality trait use projection to protect themselves from their inner rage (KS)

121. The term used to describe the frustration of the emotional needs and wishes that patients may have in relation to the analyst is:

a. Analyst as mirror

b. Counter-transference

c. The principle of evenly suspended attention

d. The rule of abstinence

e. Transference (KS)

122. In which stage of psychoanalysis does transference emerge?

a. 1

b. 2

c. 3

d. 4

e. 5 (KS)

123. The supportive techniques of psychoanalytic therapy include all of the following except the:

a. Evocative

b. Relationship-oriented

c. Repressed

d. Suggestive

e. Suppressive (KS)

124. Which of the following is an indication for insight-oriented psychotherapy?

a. Meaningful object relations

b. Poor frustration tolerance

c. Poor reality testing

d. Significant ego defects of a long-term nature

e. A tenuous ability to form a therapeutic alliance (KS)

125. All of the following statements about brief focal psychotherapy are true except:

a. Its duration is up to 1 year

b. Its focus is on internal conflict present since childhood

c. Its goal is to clarify the nature of the patient's defence

d. Its selection criteria include prospective patients having the ability to think in feeling terms

e. It involves 12 treatment hours (KS)

126. Which of the following involves a cognitive profile that includes an inflated view of self, experience and the future?

    a. Anxiety disorder

    b. Conversion disorder

    c. Depressive disorder

    d. Hypomanic disorder

    e. Paranoid personality disorder (KS)

127. Which of the following is the part of cognitive therapy that involves explaining the cognitive triad, schemas and faulty logic to the patient?

    a. Eliciting automatic thoughts

    b. Didactic aspects

    c. Identifying maladaptive assumptions

    d. Testing automatic thoughts

    e. Testing the validity of maladaptive assumptions (KS)

128. In hypnosis, which of the following is the ability to reduce peripheral awareness, resulting in greater focal attention?

    a. Absorption

    b. Dissociation

    c. Response attentiveness

    d. Suggestibility

    e. Trance development (KS)

129. All of the following are non-verbal behavioural components of social skills training except:

a. Facial expression

b. Eye contact

c. Paralinguistic features

d. Posture

e. Proxemics (KS)

130. Which of the following statements about the phases of interpersonal psychotherapy is true?

a. Three sessions are dedicated to the initial phase

b. The initial phase involves the identification of areas and warning signs of anticipated future difficulty

c. Relating issues about psychiatric symptoms to the interpersonal problem area is part of the intermediate stage

d. Reviewing significant relationships in the past and present is a component of the intermediate phase

e. Sessions 10 to 15 constitute the termination phase (KS)

Answers

Paper 1

1. d	2. e	3. e	4. a	5. c	6. a	7. e
8. e	9. d	10. b	11. c	12. a	13. a	14. e
15. c	16. e	17. d	18. c	19. a	20. e	21. b
22. b	23. e	24. a	25. c	26. b	27. b	28. e
29. d	30. a	31. e	32. c	33. a	34. e	35. c
36. d	37. d	38. e	39. c	40. e	41. b	42. a
43. d	44. a	45. a	46. c	47. a	48. d	49. a
50. c	51. c	52. a	53. a	54. e	55. c	56. d
57. a	58. e	59. d	60. d	61. a	62. c	63. e
64. b	65. b	66. c	67. a	68. d	69. c	70. e
71. e	72. a	73. b	74. e	75. a	76. c	77. d
78. d	79. c	80. c	81. e	82. e	83. a	84. d
85. c	86. c	87. b	88. e	89. a	90. c	91. d
92. d	93. a	94. e	95. b	96. b	97. a	98. b
99. d	100. c	101. d	102. c	103. c	104. d	105. e
106. e	107. a	108. c	109. a	110. b	111. b	112. a
113. c	114. c	115. d	116. c	117. d	118. c	119. e
120. c	121. b	122. b	123. c	124. c	125. c	126. b
127. d	128. e	129. d	130. d			

Paper 2

1. c	2. d	3. b	4. e	5. e	6. e	7. b
8. e	9. e	10. a	11. b	12. e	13. e	14. b
15. d	16. b	17. a	18. a	19. b	20. e	21. e
22. c	23. a	24. a	25. c	26. c	27. e	28. d
29. d	30. b	31. b	32. a	33. e	34. a	35. e
36. d	37. b	38. e	39. e	40. c	41. e	42. e
43. e	44. b	45. d	46. b	47. e	48. b	49. a
50. a	51. c	52. c	53. b	54. e	55. d	56. c
57. e	58. b	59. d	60. c	61. e	62. d	63. b
64. d	65. c	66. e	67. a	68. a	69. a	70. a
71. d	72. b	73. d	74. e	75. e	76. b	77. a
78. e	79. c	80. c	81. d	82. c	83. a	84. d
85. b	86. c	87. a	88. e	89. a	90. a	91. e
92. c	93. e	94. a	95. d	96. a	97. b	98. a
99. a	100. b	101. b	102. b	103. e	104. b	105. b
106. e	107. e	108. d	109. e	110. e	111. c	112. b
113. a	114. b	115. b	116. d	117. a	118. c	119. c
120. a	121. b	122. b	123. d	124. a	125. c	126. c
127. e	128. d	129. d	130. c			

Paper 3

1. a	2. e	3. c	4. d	5. b	6. c	7. e
8. a	9. e	10. e	11. a	12. d	13. e	14. c
15. a	16. a	17. a	18. b	19. e	20. b	21. d
22. d	23. e	24. d	25. c	26. e	27. b	28. e
29. b	30. b	31. d	32. e	33. a	34. e	35. d
36. a	37. a	38. e	39. d	40. c	41. b	42. a
43. d	44. b	45. c	46. e	47. e	48. d	49. c
50. a	51. b	52. e	53. e	54. b	55. e	56. d
57. c	58. c	59. e	60. e	61. c	62. e	63. b
64. a	65. d	66. d	67. a	68. d	69. a	70. b
71. e	72. c	73. b	74. c	75. d	76. c	77. a
78. e	79. c	80. b	81. d	82. e	83. c	84. a
85. e	86. a	87. d	88. e	89. c	90. c	91. b
92. b	93. d	94. d	95. b	96. d	97. b	98. a
99. e	100. e	101. b	102. d	103. d	104. a	105. e
106. e	107. b	108. e	109. d	110. d	111. d	112. a
113. b	114. a	115. b	116. b	117. c	118. d	119. e
120. b	121. a	122. a	123. d	124. b	125. d	126. a
127. d	128. b	129. c	130. e			

Paper 4

1. d	2. c	3. a	4. c	5. b	6. c	7. d
8. d	9. c	10. e	11. d	12. b	13. c	14. c
15. c	16. c	17. e	18. a	19. e	20. c	21. b
22. d	23. d	24. c	25. e	26. c	27. e	28. c
29. d	30. e	31. a	32. b	33. c	34. c	35. b
36. c	37. d	38. e	39. c	40. a	41. b	42. c
43. d	44. e	45. a	46. a	47. b	48. e	49. c
50. e	51. e	52. d	53. a	54. d	55. b	56. a
57. a	58. e	59. d	60. d	61. d	62. b	63. c
64. c	65. b	66. e	67. e	68. b	69. e	70. b
71. d	72. e	73. b	74. b	75. b	76. e	77. d
78. d	79. b	80. b	81. e	82. d	83. e	84. a
85. b	86. c	87. b	88. c	89. b	90. e	91. d
92. b	93. d	94. e	95. a	96. c	97. a	98. c
99. b	100. e	101. c	102. d	103. c	104. c	105. b
106. d	107. d	108. b	109. b	110. b	111. d	112. d
113. e	114. e	115. b	116. e	117. d	118. b	119. e
120. e	121. c	122. e	123. b	124. a	125. b	126. d
127. e	128. d	129. a	130. b			

Paper 5

1. a	2. b	3. c	4. d	5. c	6. a	7. b
8. a	9. a	10. b	11. c	12. b	13. b	14. b
15. e	16. b	17. a	18. b	19. b	20. b	21. d
22. d	23. a	24. d	25. e	26. e	27. a	28. e
29. d	30. c	31. a	32. a	33. a	34. c	35. e
36. e	37. d	38. b	39. a	40. b	41. b	42. c
43. e	44. c	45. e	46. d	47. d	48. d	49. b
50. a	51. a	52. b	53. b	54. c	55. c	56. c
57. d	58. d	59. c	60. e	61. b	62. c	63. c
64. d	65. a	66. e	67. e	68. d	69. c	70. e
71. e	72. b	73. e	74. e	75. e	76. b	77. c
78. c	79. c	80. b	81. e	82. d	83. d	84. b
85. b	86. b	87. b	88. e	89. b	90. d	91. d
92. e	93. e	94. b	95. a	96. d	97. a	98. c
99. d	100. e	101. e	102. a	103. e	104. c	105. c
106. e	107. e	108. b	109. c	110. b	111. c	112. b
113. e	114. c	115. b	116. d	117. b	118. d	119. b
120. c	121. d	122. b	123. a	124. a	125. e	126. d
127. b	128. a	129. c	130. c			

Index